To Sherry—

On the Road to
you're ~~on~~ in the fast lane.
Enjoy!
Be Well—
Nancie Barwick

Unstuff Yourself:

Finding Joy on the Road to Wellness

Nancie M. Barwick, DCH

Published in the United States by
Hypnotherapy Works Press

Dedication

In memory of four amazingly strong, intelligent, and unconditionally loving women who willingly shared their wisdom with me.

Rose Altshuler	April 1873–January 1971
Betty Geller	January 1907–October 2000
Jeannette Sheinfeld	February 1914–December 1993
Doreen Barwick	January 1918–February 1996

Acknowledgements

My very deep appreciation goes to Kim McGarghan for her skillful and thoughtful editing of this book, as well as her helpful suggestions. I am grateful to Patti Conklin for suggesting that this book should exist, and that I should be the one to write it. Thanks to Ken Elliott for the beautiful cover art and design. Barbara Brooker, at whose home my son was almost born, thanks for the indexing and so much more. Many thanks to my mother, Mimi Geller, for her assistance with final review and her valuable suggestions.

I want to acknowledge my many friends, colleagues and clients who have greeted the news of this book with such kindness and interest.

As always, I am indebted to my husband, Tim, and children, Johannah and Samuel, for their love and support as I got rid of my stuff and then as I worked on this book. I thank my parents and siblings for being who they are, the perfect family for me to become who I am.

Foreword

by Patti Conklin

There are a few people in this world that continually shock and surprise us. Nancie is one of these people. She is an individual who has faced many challenges in her life yet has always remained joyful and optimistic. Having known her for over 5 years, I've sat and watched her growth, awareness, eloquence, optimism, intelligence and overall joy. What a great adventure she has been on!

Having met Nancie while she was in the midst of her disease of Muscular Dystrophy, I was delighted by her optimism for life and work. What a phenomenal teacher and practitioner she is! Being in her scooter never ever slowed her down. I have watched her lecture at many conferences throughout the years, I have had the honor of being in her home town as a guest speaker, but most of all, I've gotten to know Nancie as a human being, and what an incredible human being she is. Now, I delight in seeing Nancie popping out of chairs, running up and down stairs, riding bicycles, no longer needing her faithful scooter.

In this book, you will find her awareness, love, intelligence, humor (LOTS of humor) but most of all, Nancie is able to put her thoughts in "everyday speak" which can be a very challenging task. She has insights that most of us can only begin to grasp.

Over the years I've watched Nancie in her scooter, never slowing down. I always felt as though when she was ready to let go of her disability she would let me know. I never offered her help as many had done. It is clear to me that when people are ready to heal they find the right facilitator for them. I can't express the peace I felt when Nancie approached me in February of 2003 and stated that it was time for us to work together. I do a process called "Cellular Cleansing," which I developed over the years. It is a synthesis of Hypnosis, Neuro-Linguistic Programming and my energy. Nancie traveled with her scooter to Atlanta on April 7th. Two days later, she was walking, no scooter, no cane, no support. By April 20th, she had tucked away her "disability equipment" for good.

Enjoy this journey with a wonderful human being who has been to both ends of the health spectrum and has enjoyed life all the way!

Patti L. Conklin, M.Ht
Medical Intuitive

Contents

Introduction

For a large number of people, the search for wellness is a lifelong quest. There are hundreds of books and tapes full of good information about ways to engage in this search. Most of these methods contain useful and fulfilling ideas, and a few even tell the reader how to know when wellness is found. Struggle in the cause of achieving wellness is generally recommended, with changes in diet and lifestyle being required, like it or not. Little is said about the need for joy in this process.

However, if we are going to achieve true wellness, most of us need to unstuff our lives and increase the joy we experience on a daily basis. Truly well people are joyful, not in a false, out-of-control, or frenetic way but in a real, honest, and fulfilling way that is quietly easy to sustain. It is so easy precisely because it is real.

To unstuff our lives we need to remove the old tapes, false information, incorrect learning, beliefs that no longer serve us, and other bits of fluff and nonsense that currently fill our psyches and consciousness. We need to determine what we need to keep and what must go. Comfortably removing all the stuff requires readiness and preparation, so that we are able to let it go without a fight. When we are ready and fully prepared to let go of our stuff, the letting-go is a joyful experience in itself.

In some traditions and healing methodologies, the goal is to remove everything unique to that person so that the individual becomes bland and free of personal idiosyncrasies. Nothing could be further from the truth! As you remove your harmful stuff, you will be finding your true joy. That is your INDIVIDUAL joy, what really gets you happy and excited. If anything, people who are truly unstuffed and well are more who they are, more individual than ever before, and certainly more so than their friends and neighbors, who are still full of stuff and without their true joy. Your idiosyncrasies will remain as long as they bring you joy; those which do not please you, or even cause you harm, will simply fall away.

While this is really a book for you, at times it is about me. Personal stories can be great convincers. I was born with muscular dystrophy. I had that condition as a part of my experience until I was 44 years old. At that point, and with the help of a wise facilitator, I was able to remove it. I was ready to get rid of the stuff that was holding the muscular dystrophy in my body, and had thoroughly prepared to unstuff myself completely. After my experience, I decided to assist others in making these types of changes.

Now, you may not have a serious medical condition like the one I did, or maybe you do, it makes no difference. The process is the same and the results are extremely beneficial, even if there is no medical concern at this time. Often our stuff merely makes us less happy than we would otherwise be, less fulfilled or "stuck" in unhealthy patterns. Sometimes it makes us sick, and sometimes it makes us miserable. It never makes us happy or well. Once we are able to let it all go, there is room for whatever makes us truly joyful.

What Is Wellness?

We have all heard of Wellness; there are Wellness Centers, Wellness classes, and a myriad of books on Wellness. We all want to be well, whatever that is. We think it might be the opposite of sick, so is it the absence of illness? Can a positive goal be the absence of something else?

Wellness is not the absence of something else; it is a positive in its own right. Simply put, Wellness is that which completes the individual so that he or she can truly feel right and good in himself or herself. For some people this means a physical healing from illness or disease. For others, it is a mental or spiritual sense of comfort and well-being. For many, it is a little of both, or even a lot of both.

Well people need not be perfect physically, mentally, or emotionally. They need not be in a spiritual place that others would define as correct. Well people still live in physical human bodies that can be injured or even disabled, though amazing healings can and do take place on the physical plane. Well people have the intellect they were born to have, and may or may not be mentally skilled. Well people experience human emotions—how flat life would be without love, joy, wonder, and—yes—even sadness and anger when appropriate. The real difference is that well people do not allow these emotions to overwhelm them, or to short-circuit their electrical systems. They stay reasonably grounded.

Let's look at physical wellness for a moment. After all, we all live in physical bodies and we know what physical wellness is. At least we think we do!

Physical wellness means that the person's body is as healthy as it is possible for that body to be. A physically well person is comfortable in his or her own skin, feeling reasonably comfortable with its shape and size even when there is a desire for change in this area. When we are well physically, our body functions in a way that supports our ability to live and do the things we choose to do. It is not about perfection as others see it. It is about comfort and function that is appropriate for us at this time in our life.

Most of us view a young, strong body that is without obvious disfigurement or damage to be the epitome of wellness. In a sense this is true, certainly the medical profession would consider this individual well. Of course, the young, strong person may be truly well, but he may also be quite unwell. It might be the person next door, elderly and frail, who is truly well.

Physical wellness is simply the optimal state of health for the body as it was made and at the age it is. Will a 44-year-old woman who is 5'4" ever be a 22-year-old 6' supermodel? No, of course not. Can this woman be truly well? Absolutely! While it is possible to change the present and the future, the past has already happened. It is, however, possible and beneficial to change our perception of the past so that it can no longer limit us.

Mental wellness and emotional wellness are the states of mind and thought where we are most comfortable. They are states wherein the individual is able to cope with the incidents that happen in the course of a normal life without allowing his or her own inner peace to be compromised.

When a person is mentally and emotionally well, he or she is not in a state of unawareness or complete calm at all times. We all live in the real world; sometimes things happen which displease us, and sometimes we experience emotions that are unpleasant. This is normal, and a part of a rich and varied life. For a person who is emotionally or mentally unwell, these events can be unsettling or even cause severe distress. However, when someone is well both mentally and emotionally, he or she does not feel as completely out of control and will recover more quickly if he or she experiences some upset. A person in a state of true mental and emotional wellness is able to realize that they are not harmed by the words and actions of others but rather by their own reactions to them.

Often, other people say and do things we do not want them to, either in their own lives or with regard to us. They may tell us that we are doing something wrong or even that our beliefs and lifestyle are bad. Depending on our relationship to the person, we may feel upset by these types of statements, which are often perceived as attacks. However, it is important to realize that these statements can and should have no effect whatsoever on who we are or what we choose for ourselves. Once we are in a state of mental and emotional wellness, we are able to observe the actions or words of others without taking them on. When we are well we are strong enough to hold onto our own selves regardless of what is going on around us.

We also need to recognize that the things others do in their own lives have no effect on us. Even when our children make what we might consider to be poor choices in their relationships, work, education or other important parts of their lives, we need to understand clearly that these are their life choices, not ours. Our dearest loved ones are on their own paths and, while we may walk alongside them for a time, we are not on their paths and they are not on ours. Each individual is living the life he or she is living and we are all ultimately responsible only for and to ourselves. In a state of Wellness, it is more possible to make these distinctions.

Regardless of an individual's belief system, everyone has a spiritual side. For many individuals, the spiritual aspects of life can be a less-than-comfortable state for them to experience. Those people might believe that they are spiritually unwell, and they might be looking for a sense of wellness in their spiritual lives. This is an excellent opportunity to explore spiritual practices which might be enriching and supportive for that individual. However, this needs to be taken on an individual basis and the only one who will know if the new practices are appropriate is the individual involved.

We are not talking about religious practice or belief, which is an intensely personal issue and not within the scope of this book. People can be spiritually well whatever their religious belief system, in fact, even if they have no religious belief system. Atheism, Buddhism, Christianity,

Hinduism, Judaism, Islam, Paganism, Satanism, Wicca and every other belief system are absolutely equal in this regard as long as it works for the individual.

What is spiritual wellness, then? To be well spiritually is to be engaging regularly in spiritual practices that offer the individual a sense of ease and completeness in his or her own soul or spirit, no matter what that means to that person. It means that the person is satisfied and feels enriched in some way by these practices. Just about everyone engages in spiritual practices, regardless of their belief or lack of belief in spirit. Spiritual practices can include, but are not limited to, music, art, reading, meditation, prayer, chanting, yoga, or even just staring into a fire. It makes no difference what spiritual practice an individual chooses, even if it is not a part of the tradition in which they were raised. It must feed their individual spirit, whatever they sense that to be.

Wellness sounds wonderful, but many believe it is unattainable for them. Nothing could be further from the truth. Regardless of who you are and what your situation might be, you can be well if you will follow the **Simple Steps to Wellness** we will discuss later.

How Do I Know If I Am Well?

It is very easy to determine if you are well. Physical, Mental, Emotional, and Spiritual Wellness are all parts of being well and all must be addressed in order to determine if you are well. It is true that many of the determining factors are subjective, but of course Wellness is often a matter of individual perception.

1. Is my physical body healthy? Y/N
2. Am I comfortable with my physical situation? Y/N
3. Does my body function as I would want it to? Y/N
4. Do I stay calm when life events are upsetting? Y/N
5. Do I regain my calm within a reasonable time after an upsetting event? Y/N
6. When others criticize me, do I refuse to allow it to affect me deeply? Y/N
7. Regardless of what another may say or do, am I able to understand that it is his or her own path or issue and in no way related to me? Y/N
8. Do I engage in enriching spiritual practices? Y/N
9. Do I experience a sense of ease in my spirit? Y/N
10. Do my practices allow me to feel complete in myself? Y/N

If you answered "no" to any of these questions, you may not be as well in that area as you would like to be. The more "no" answers you have, the more you may have issues with wellness in a number of areas. Please remember that this quiz is intended to assist you in determining if you are indeed well or if this is an issue you need to consider in your own life.

Why Wellness?

Why is Wellness desirable? When we are well, our physical, mental, emotional, and spiritual bodies are in the most appropriate condition for us at that time. We are able to live our lives the way we choose to live them, enjoying all the good things that life has to offer. We can contribute our best to the world around us. We can care for our families more effectively. Whatever Wellness means to us, it is a positive thing.

When we are in a state of Wellness, our troubles seem to be less troublesome. We are better able to cope with whatever we are experiencing, regardless of the situation. We may still dislike a situation or want to change it, but we can do so more effectively and efficiently. We may even fail at something we attempt to do; after all, we are human. However, we can deal with that failure more comfortably and we can adjust our actions more competently so that we are less likely to fail in any future attempt. At least we will not fail in the same way.

As we have seen, Wellness is a comfortable and pleasant place to be.

Where is the City of Wellness?

The City of Wellness is not a geographical location. It is the metaphor that we are using for the state of being well. The City of Wellness is within each of us. It is the ideal that we all have of being well, regardless of our current degree of wellness.

The Roads to the City of Wellness are a metaphorical name we use to describe the various modalities, methodologies, and ways of getting to the City. In other words, the roads are the actions we take to increase our wellness. These roads can be therapies, techniques, things we do for ourselves, or things that others do for (or to) us to increase our wellness. Just like in real travel, some of the roads are better for some types of vehicles, some are faster, and some are closed or have detours. It is up to the individual to choose the best road for the conditions.

Stuff—What Stuff?

So, what is this "stuff" of which we speak? We have worked on ourselves, been Rolfed, regressed, and rebirthed. We have twisted our beliefs into knots in therapy or listening to "healers" who tell us the ONE TRUE way to serenity or whatever they are calling it. However, we still have our issues, our problems have not really gone away. The reason for the lack of total success is that our stuff is still there.

So, what is this stuff anyway? Simply put, stuff consists of the old messages, old ideas, and old ways of thinking and doing that no longer serve us. It's the ideas we learned in childhood, the "I can't" messages we give ourselves every day that we first heard at our mother's knee. It's the mean things our first-grade teacher said when we had trouble learning to read fluently or what the school bully did or said that we turned into beliefs in our own minds. It's whatever happened in our lives to make us feel "less than" or unworthy.

All people have some stuff regardless of how idyllic their childhood may have been or how loving their family. There is no blame to be laid on anyone necessarily for our stuff. Some young children learn to put the stuff on themselves, pushing their limits in school or sports and becoming nervous, anxious little people in the process. You may have failed on a test or even a whole subject, so you decided you were stupid, even though it is not true. That's stuff too.

All of this stuff is moving around in the body and mind. Maybe we replay an uncomfortable experience over and over *ad nauseum,* which literally means until illness. It makes us sick. Replay illnesses tend to be emotional stuckness, Obsessive Compulsive Disorder, anxiety, upset stomachs and sleep deprivation illnesses.

Sometimes we don't replay a particular scene or event, at least not that we can identify. We might re-experience distress in situations that are similar to the one that caused the original bit of stuff in an area of the body. Every time we encounter a situation or even a person that reminds our unconscious mind of the origin of the stuff, we may become more uncomfortable. In many cases, these bits of stuff can reach critical mass and cause an illness, disease, or pain. Critical mass illnesses tend to be muscular or joint conditions, TMJ (Temporal Mandibular Joint) Syndrome, masses, lumps, etc.

Most people have both of these types of stuff in their body. Sometimes we replay and sometimes we do not. There is also a third type of stuff that can be going on in the body. This is a free-floating type, which does not replay or make us anxious in certain situations. It is simply there and, if left to its own devices, will rub an area raw before moving on. It's that nagging feeling that something is not quite right in our world. This stuff tends to lead to anger, frustration at small things, depression and other unpleasant emotions. There are only two real human emotions, Love and Fear, and this stuff is really Fear. It's the unnamed fears of childhood and the fears that perhaps we don't like to admit as adults just floating around in our body. This sort of stuff weakens the immune system, fatigues the body, and puts strain on the vital organs including the brain.

All of these types of stuff occur naturally for human beings because of events that happen as we go through our lives. They can certainly be caused by terrible events, but the precipitating events need not be awful or enormous. Regardless of the cause or type, our stuff does not contribute to our joy and can even block our experience of it. Therefore, it must be reduced and removed as much as possible.

Working with Replay Stuff

Replay stuff is the stuff we get from replaying unpleasant experiences repeatedly. Often the replay takes place while we sleep, so that it reruns in our dreams and plays on the inside of our eyelids during times we are unaware of dreaming. Sometimes it replays on a subconscious level while we are awake, like a murmur we can't quite hear.

The original experience might have been horrible, such as children's experiences of abuse. It can also have been mildly unpleasant, which most of us have experienced such as giving a wrong answer at school. It really makes no difference, the important issue with replay stuff is that an unpleasant experience happened and the individual's unconscious mind revisits it and revives the experience and feelings.

Most people have experienced replay from time to time, though people who are well tend to throw it off fairly quickly. Some people have a little bit of replay stuff that stays around for a while, but not long enough to cause permanent difficulties. However, it can easily grow to a level where it does cause problems if it is allowed to remain. The individual who has replay stuff-caused illness or difficulty is not to be blamed. It is not that they are weak or foolish in any way. It is simply that the amount of replay they are experiencing has overwhelmed their body's ability to remove it.

Replay stuff-related illnesses can include sleeplessness. You may be really tired from lack of sleep. It is easy to understand how the constant replay of unpleasant scenes whenever the person falls asleep could tend to make sleeping difficult. People who do not get enough sleep become nervous and jumpy. They can make poor decisions, which can cause more difficulties in their lives in terms of work, interpersonal relationships, and decision-making.

Sleeplessness can cause other medical problems, including Fibromyalgia, a medical condition that is characterized by pain, fatigue, and, sometimes, mental confusion. Fibromyalgia is reaching epidemic proportions in this society at this time. Researchers have proven a link between lack of sufficient restful sleep and the development of Fibromyalgia. In several medical studies, healthy volunteers were deprived of sufficient deep, restful sleep for a period of several weeks. They developed symptoms of Fibromyalgia within three weeks. When they were again allowed to sleep as deeply as they wanted or needed to, they all recovered quickly. Replay stuff can cause this condition because we may replay in our sleep to the extent that we are not getting good rest at night. For many people, the restoration of restful sleep patterns can eradicate any symptoms of Fibromyalgia.

Replay stuff causes anxiety, Obsessive-Compulsive Disorder (OCD), and similar issues. This is partly because of the lack of restful sleep and partly due to the replay that occurs just below awareness in a waking state. Even if we are not aware of the replay that is going on, the result of it is often these types of conditions that we feel we cannot control. The constant replaying of unpleasant events, even though it is unconscious, naturally makes us anxious. Often people who experience anxiety express a feeling of being out of control, which fuels their anxiety even more. They attempt to control whatever aspects of their world that they feel they can control, often using odd behavior that seems to them to help them to be in better control of their world. They can become obsessive or compulsive in their insistence that this behavior must occur.

It is certainly understandable when we consider that the replay stuff keeps the person from sleeping which makes them anxious. In an attempt to quell the anxiety, the person works at controlling whatever they can. They can become quite rigid in their insistence that they control these parts of their world, to the extent that their behavior can be perceived by others as irrational and annoying, even crazy.

The anxious behavior often results in job loss or social stigmatization, which results in more upset and anxious feelings due to financial stress or a feeling of not being able to make life work. People who experience this type of distress are often diagnosed with mental illnesses, which results in more stigmatization.

It is unfortunate that those individuals who have a great deal of replay stuff-created anxiety have to deal with social stigmatization. When a person is socially stigmatized, that means that he or she is not included in the mainstream of social activities because whatever trait or characteristic or behavior he or she seems to have is not valued by society. Sometimes it is even considered a negative trait to such an extent that people are uncomfortable with that person. For example, some people become so anxious that they develop ideas of what will keep them safe, and those things can be wearing the same clothing or hoarding items that most people would consider to be garbage. Some folks feel safer if they perform certain acts in the same order or in the same way on a regular basis. These acts are called rituals. Some rituals intrude on the comfort or freedom of others by forcing them to witness bizarre behavior or not to touch certain items, etc. Most members of society avoid spending time with people who would intrude on them in that way, so the individual is stigmatized or isolated by society. Even long-term friends and family members can become unwilling to be with a person whose anxious behavior makes them uncomfortable.

Due to the unconscious replay of distressing material, excessive stomach acid or activity can occur. This can lead to upset stomachs, diarrhea and, if left to its own devices, Irritable Bowel Syndrome (IBS) or ulcers. These painful and often debilitating conditions can result in lifelong disability.

IBS is a very unpleasant condition that is very difficult to treat medically. People with this condition can suffer from any or all of these symptoms: constipation, diarrhea, bloating, gas, pain, and nausea. Some individuals discover that certain foods trigger their symptoms and others seem to feel ill no matter what they eat or drink. IBS is often terribly limiting to the life of the individual because they do not feel well a lot of the time, they may need to be near a restroom at all times and they may not be able to work or attend school. In fact, IBS is the second most frequent reason for missed days from work in the United States, after respiratory illness such as colds and flu.

Ulcers are sores or holes in the lining of the stomach or other parts of the digestive system. While the latest research seems to indicate that ulcers may be caused by a virus or other external agent, excessive intestinal acidity is implicated in their severity. When there is too much acid in the immediate environment of the ulcer, it is less likely that the ulcer will heal. It is also more likely that the initial injury to the digestive lining will be irritated and become more severe or chronic. Diet modifications in conjunction with acid-reducing medications and lifestyle changes can certainly help to reduce the severity of ulcers and even to help them to heal. However, removing the stuff that makes the person anxious will usually reduce the amount of acidity permanently to the degree to which it was increased by the anxiety in the first place.

We have discovered that replay stuff leads to significant suffering and discomfort. As we replay the distressing situations or messages over and over we increase the amount of stuff in the area of the body where that type of stuff sits for us, increasing the chance of illness or anchoring and intensifying the illness if it has already appeared. This means that we continue to get sicker and suffer increasingly the longer we allow the replay to continue.

It is important to note, however, that there is no blame or fault in replay stuff or in any of our stuff in fact. We take on the stuff we take on unconsciously, and do not consciously choose it. Some people believe that we make these choices to set up life lessons we need to learn, probably before we came to this lifetime. It is possibly true that on a soul level, we may choose to take on certain stuff and hold it in certain places in the body; certainly many people believe this to be true. However, these choices are not made consciously. Even if this is true, they were not chosen consciously, and we have no way of knowing why the soul made the choice it did. It is important to understand this point very clearly because it is of no benefit to assign blame to an individual who is dealing with the results of this stuff, illness and disease.

How Do I Determine If I Have Replay Stuff?

Now that we have discussed and defined Replay Stuff, it is useful to determine whether this type of stuff exists in your life and what, if any, conditions it may be causing. The following checklist may be helpful as long as you answer it honestly.

1. Is my sleep often disturbed? Y/N
2. Do I have difficulty waking up? Y/N
3. Do I fall asleep during the day? Y/N
4. If I don't actually have the opportunity to fall asleep, do I want to? Y/N
5. Do I have vague feelings of dread? Y/N
6. Does my anxiety interfere with my life? Y/N
7. Does my behavior upset others? Y/N

8. Do I use rituals to manage my anxiety? Y/N

9. Do I have pain and other symptoms when I don't sleep well? Y/N

10. When I feel anxious, do my stomach or intestines react? Y/N

If you answered "yes" to any question, you might have replay stuff that is causing you difficulties. The more "yes" answers, the more likely it is that you have this type of stuff. Even if you are not consciously aware of the origins of the replay stuff, you can address it in order to loosen and remove it.

So, how do we work with replay stuff so that it loosens? There are a number of variables to consider. The individual dealing with the replay stuff is the only one able to make this decision, even if he or she does not seem to know at first. Some of this stuff is close enough to the surface that we can access it consciously by thinking and talking about it. Some of it is so deeply buried that this is not possible, no matter how hard we try.

Is the stuff close enough to the consciousness to address it in Cognitive-Behavioral Therapy, talk therapy, or similar modalities? In order to work with it in these modalities, the individual must know what the original events were, and how the stuff is manifesting in their mind, either as replay during sleep or on a subtle level while the person is awake. If this is the case, these modalities can be immensely useful in preparing the stuff to depart. Be aware, however, that while they seldom remove it completely, they definitely loosen its hold so that further work is possible and comfortable. They also provide some control over the resulting problematic behavior at times, because the person is able to recognize the behavior that is causing difficulty in his life and then control this behavior on a conscious level. These modalities also offer a degree of understanding of the reason for the unsettling behavior. For many individuals, this control and understanding can be beneficial in preparing to release the stuff.

If the stuff is below the surface of consciousness, as is so often the case, all the talk therapy and behavioral therapy in the world will not affect it. It is not available to the conscious mind. In those situations, hypnotherapy may well be useful in loosening the stuff. If it is really deeply embedded, the techniques of Time Line Therapy™, Emotional Freedom Technique (EFT), or similar modalities can be used to good effect. These and other techniques will be described and explained later, in the section on Loosening Techniques.

However, regardless of the depth of the stuff, there are things you can do at home on a daily basis to begin to loosen your own replay stuff. If you are aware of the replay, that is, if it is available to your own conscious mind you can reframe it. This means that when the situation comes up in your mind you can rewrite it. If, for example, your mother called you fat and stupid on your fifth birthday, you can imagine her simply wishing you a happy birthday. You might have to do this several hundred times consciously in the first few days, but over time it will begin to replace the original version in your replay and will become a benign memory that you will not have to replay any more.

With unconscious replays, you can have equally wonderful results with another simple technique. Let's imagine, for example, that you wake up every morning with an upset stomach and a headache from clenching your jaws. Chances are there is some unconscious replay stuff going on. You may have no conscious idea of what you are replaying on the insides of your eyelids every night, but you can still reframe it. Every night before going to sleep, have a nice relaxing hot beverage such as chamomile tea or whatever you enjoy as long as it contains no caffeine or alcohol or other stimulant. You may want to have a hot/warm bath with Epsom Salt before bed, as this releases toxins and tends to encourage restful sleep. Get into your bed in a comfortable position and imagine pleasant things as you drift off to a deep, restful sleep. These will vary from individual to individual, but some popular visualizations include favorite places in nature, successful experiences you have had or plan to have in the future, and favorite people in your life.

A good way to track the success of these techniques is to keep a journal. Write down how you are feeling on a daily basis. Include dreams, random associations, experiences, emotions, and physical sensations. If you do this for a period of 21 days, you will have a good record of how the replay stuff is loosening. However, you do not have to stop after 21 days; in fact, you should not stop if there is any residual replay stuff left even after you begin to work with it therapeutically.

As you begin to reduce the hold of your replay stuff, you will probably begin to sleep more deeply and restfully. The more good sleep you get, the better you are likely to feel naturally. The better you feel, the more energetic you may become, which will assist you as you move forward toward removing your stuff permanently.

Working with Critical Mass Stuff

The second major type of stuff we carry is "Critical Mass" stuff. Critical mass stuff is usually caused by unpleasant experiences that take place often in the person's life. However, it can also be caused by strong emotions, which recur in similar situations throughout a person's life. Each time the individual has either the experience or the emotion, more stuff is created. This stuff is not replayed every night but sits in a particular area of the body, building and building until it reaches a size and density (or critical mass) that enables it to cause damage to the organ, system, or tissues in which it sits. This is why it is known as "Critical Mass" stuff.

Very often, family, friends, and colleagues will consider the individual who is dealing with Critical Mass stuff to be very nice, but that person has achieved this by stashing his or her true feelings into whatever part of the body he or she first used to store that emotion or feeling. It is an unconscious behavior that often starts as a defense mechanism. If a child discovers that the expression of a true emotion is unsafe, then a wise child would stash the emotion somewhere in the body. The individual ends up stashing so much stuff into an area that it is unable to hold it in a healthy way and a disease process starts. Of course, no one does this consciously. It happens on an unconscious level, and there is no conscious choice about stashing the stuff in a particular place or, indeed, stashing it in the body at all.

Diseases such as muscular dystrophy, arthritis, lupus, polymyalgia rheumatica, cancer, TMJ (Temporal Mandibular Joint) Syndrome, multiple sclerosis, and neurofibromas are often critical mass-related conditions. Even subcategories that appear to be hereditary are related to critical mass. What is inherited is the tendency to stash the stuff into certain areas or systems of the body. The emotion will be different for different people, but they are based in Fear.

All of the critical mass stuff-related diseases or conditions share some interesting characteristics. They are all physical illnesses that exist in specific body parts or types of tissue while the rest of the body is left untouched. They are not systemic. Rather, the specific area is not able to function properly. Whatever the diagnosis might be, it can be described as a diseased area of an otherwise healthy body. It might be a single small area such as a single tumor or a large number of small areas like neurofibromas and arthritis or the multiple lesions that occur in multiple sclerosis. It can also be a large area of the body, which we might see in muscular dystrophy or lupus.

As we can see, the Critical Mass stuff-related conditions behave exactly how we would expect a critical mass to behave. The stuff affects certain areas of the body but leaves the rest of the body untouched, though side effects of the condition may affect other areas and aspects of the individual's health. With muscular dystrophy, for example, the skeletal muscles are generally affected but the cardiac muscle is not. Certainly, the inability to exercise, medications, and other results of the muscular dystrophy can affect the heart or any other part of the body that is normal. However, the actual disorder did not cause this problem in itself.

Diseases that show up in young children can also be critical mass-based, but the building of the mass began before birth with the emotions of the mother and father during the development of the egg and the sperm, and with the emotions of the mother during her pregnancy. In her excellent book, ***Molecules of Emotion,*** Dr. Candace Pert describes how emotions create chemicals called peptides in the body, and how these chemicals can either contribute to or detract from health. Like most chemicals in the mother's body, these peptides can probably pass through the placenta into a baby's bloodstream and therefore into the baby's body. It is thought that these peptides can also be present in minute amounts in the sperm and/or the egg, ending up in the baby's body that way. There is no way to prove or disprove this theory at this time.

Again, it is important to note that there is no blame or fault to be found here. The parents did not intentionally feel fear-based emotions before the baby's birth, and they certainly never consciously intended to make their child ill. They did not intentionally send the stuff into the baby's body to do harm, though that is what happened. They would certainly have avoided doing this damage if they could have done so.

When a child develops or is born with a medical condition or disability, parents often respond with a guilt emotion, which sits in their body and can build to the point of illness. This is why we so often see serious illness developing in the parents of children with disabilities or illnesses. This is not helpful because it is the child's unconscious mind, not the parents' behavior, which stashes the stuff in a specific place in the body and continues to stash it there. It is understandable that the parents would feel guilty, especially if they perceive that their emotions or actions (smoking, for example) caused the child's illness. They really need to understand that they did not consciously give their child the building blocks of the medical issues they now face, and that they can accept no blame for it. The best thing these loving parents can do is to receive whatever form of counseling and help they prefer for these feelings before they become the building blocks for a critical mass of their own. In order to help their child as much as possible, parents need to take care of their own needs and remain as healthy as they can.

How Do I Determine if I Have Critical Mass Stuff

This checklist is intended to help individuals discover whether they have significant Critical Mass Stuff or not. Please use it to assist you in answering that question for yourself. Remember that a checklist is only the first step in learning about your own situation and dealing with it.

1. Have I had a number of similar unpleasant experiences and/or emotions in my life? Y/N

2. Do I react with strong emotion when

I am reminded of the above? Y/N

3. Do I experience increased physical symptoms in some situations? Y/N

4. Do any symptoms increase when I feel certain emotions? Y/N

5. Do I have any health problem in my muscles, such as weakness or fatigue? Y/N

6. Do I have any health issues with organs, nerves, or bones? Y/N

7. Do I experience lumps or growths of any type? Y/N

8. Was I born with a medical diagnosis or disability? Y/N

9. Is there a supposed genetic predisposition to a medical issue? Y/N

10. Did I develop a health issue after my child's disability was diagnosed? Y/N

If you answered "yes" to any question, you could well be dealing with Critical Mass stuff. The more "yes" answers you have, the more likely it is that you are dealing with this type of stuff to some degree. You can use this information as a starting point for working with this stuff.

As we have seen, Critical Mass stuff causes conditions that are characterized by significant pain and often a degree of disability. What can we do about it? There are really two issues to address. The first is the result of the stuff that is the medical condition the individual is experiencing. The second is the Critical Mass stuff itself.

First, let's address the first issue, the resulting medical condition. Muscular dystrophy, arthritis, and the rest are generally characterized by pain and interruption of physical abilities. If you are experiencing these situations, pay attention to them. They are messages that the body is sending that there is a real need for help and care. Get regular massage therapy or utilize other modalities that feel right to you. Allow your body to rest. See your medical doctor if that feels right to you, but do not get caught up in the emotional roller coaster that testing and treatment can cause. Use adaptive devices as needed. Do these things with joy and gratitude for what they can do for you. Do not allow yourself to go into shame or fear regarding the use of devices or health care services. There is no reason to create another deposit of stuff. Remember that it is likely to be temporary, just until the Critical Mass stuff is gone, and that you need to give your body the care it needs to heal. Even if it were to become permanent, it is no big deal, you can be completely well and still require the use of some equipment or therapeutic services.

If the person with the medical condition is a friend or relative, remember that it is his or her stuff, not yours. What to do about it is that individual's decision, the only things that others who care about a person can do is to be lovingly supportive and give unconditional regard. If he or she makes a choice to do something you feel is incorrect, that has to be fine with you...it is not your decision. If it is a child under the age of about 15 for whom you have responsibility or guardianship, you will need to make decisions for him or her but be aware of the child's responses so that you can make the best choices for him or her. Children are on their own paths and as a parent, guardian or loving adult, your duty is to make that path possible while attending to issues the child is not able to understand at this time.

After attending to the physical situations caused by the stuff, it is time to address the stuff itself. Critical Mass often tends to relate to issues and situations whose origins we do not remember, sometimes beginning in the womb. Remember there is no blame in any sort of stuff. It simply exists.

Critical Mass Stuff is unlike replay stuff in significant ways. It does not become stronger from being revisited on a regular basis. It just sits in the body and grows as more of it is created by repeated experience of a specific emotion. It can become so large and unwieldy that the affected area of the body becomes dense and has difficulty functioning. If it sits in the muscles, for example, this can result in muscle aches or weakness. A diagnosis of muscular dystrophy or some similar illness can result. Getting rid of the critical mass stuff will, in most cases, allow the muscles to function more appropriately. Often the diagnosis is revised or removed.

Critical mass stuff is relatively easy to remove, though it is important to make sure you remove as much of it as possible and do not allow it to build up again so that you do not experience more symptoms. If the symptoms appear to be returning, the fear that is created can then sit in the body part or organ. This would tend to recreate the medical condition, which doctors would call a relapse or the end of a remission.

One effective way to loosen or even remove critical mass stuff is with the Emotional Freedom Technique or

EFT. This simple technique is used by many hypnotherapists and other therapists to reduce or remove the emotional baggage someone is carrying with regard to a specific issue. It creates an electrical circuit in the body using acupuncture meridians. As the therapist taps on the appropriate points and both therapist and client repeat certain phrases, the emotion is reduced and remains diminished. This is not to say that you will never again feel anger or whatever, but merely that you will not be as angry in a certain type of situation as you might have been in the past. You will be able to manage your feelings more effectively and therefore will not create any more stuff in that area.

Talk therapy can be useful. It certainly loosens the stuff for later removal. In addition, if the stuff is recent enough and near enough to the surface it may be removed. However, it is important to note that studies have shown that 200 hours of talk therapy results in a mere 36% change in behavior, so it is not an effective method of removing stuff and preventing its return. It is, however, very helpful in developing an intellectual understanding of the types of events and issues that create your stuff. Each individual is unique in how he or she creates and stores stuff. Often this understanding helps us to avoid getting emotionally involved in situations that cause problems for us.

In general, hypnotherapy is a wonderful way to loosen and remove a good percentage of the stuff that is clogging an area of the body. Because it bypasses the conscious mind's resistance and roadblocks, hypnosis can allow the individual who is ready to do so to release blockages that have been festering for many years.

Another wonderful modality that can assist with the reduction and loosening of critical mass stuff is massage therapy. Massage removes lactic acid from the body. The available literature on massage makes it clear that this is a major effect of this modality. Lactic acid is a waste product from the use or damage of muscle, including cardiac muscle. It can sit in the lymphatic system where it can cause illness and reduce the function of the lymph glands. It can also sit in the muscle itself, causing pain and loss of function. Therefore, its removal reduces pain. The pain might be a part of the cause of the Critical Mass stuff, in a sort of vicious circle. Stuff causes pain, which causes distress, causing more stuff. For this reason, the work of a massage therapist can often reduce this type of stuff.

Critical mass stuff can certainly create difficulties and diseases. It is very nasty stuff, created by the body and mind from the experiences and emotions of our life. It is, however, removable and therefore not permanent.

Loosening this stuff in order to make it more easy and comfortable to remove can also be fun. Massage, for example, is usually a pleasant experience and there is no reason an individual should not enjoy it. Whatever modality people choose, if they can enjoy the loosening process they will not create more stuff because of that process. They will simply have an enjoyable experience.

Working with Free-Floating Stuff

Free-floating stuff, as its name suggests, does not stay in one place building up to a critical mass. Instead, it is the bits of flotsam and jetsam that float around the body, stopping in one place or another for a time and moving on. It does not stay in any place permanently, though it may seem to revisit the same or similar areas frequently

Free-floating stuff irritates and inflames the area it visits, causing an immune system reaction and fatigue of the area. These random and frequent irritations weaken the immune system and distract it from its primary job of fighting off infectious agents. With the immune system distracted, the individual may experience more than normal frequency and severity of infection and illness. Various body systems and organs can become fatigued and even malfunction due to the effects of free-floating stuff. Sometimes the immune system reacts in unusual ways, usually overreacting, in dealing with specific agents and the individual experiences what we call an allergic reaction to that agent.

Free-floating stuff is the result of painful emotions or experiences that were infrequent or even one-time-only situations in a person's life. Generally speaking, this stuff is not caused by the big, awful, or terribly uncomfortable experiences and situations. It tends to be caused by the smaller situations that are distressing for the individual but not as much so as that which causes replay stuff. For example, we discussed that giving a wrong answer at school could potentially cause replay if it is severely uncomfortable for the person. If it is not severe enough to cause replay for that individual, yet is still pretty unpleasant, it may result in a bit of free-floating stuff. Another individual may not get any stuff from giving a wrong answer. It all depends on that person's perception of the incident.

This stuff is not as large as critical mass stuff, nor is it as well observed as replay stuff. It sort of slides in under the radar of the conscious mind, being small and very mobile. It is the stealth bomber of the body, hitting wherever it chooses without regard to the individual's wishes. Its effects can include all sorts of autoimmune disorders, weakness, fatigue, and other difficult to diagnose ailments. These effects occur due to the irritation of the various parts and systems of the body as this stuff floats throughout the whole body.

If the immune system is constantly being triggered by small irritations from free-floating stuff, it may begin to behave strangely. It may misfire because of fatigue and confusion. It may have more difficulty recognizing "self" and "dangerous other" and frequently confuse the two. If the immune system cannot tell the difference between the individual's body and things that could harm the body, it may begin to attack indiscriminately. This would be called an autoimmune disorder.

Allergies and multiple chemical sensitivities can be created by free-floating stuff as well. The immune system, overworked and confused, may begin to identify a wide variety of substances, chemicals, and foods as dangerous. Think for a moment about the soldier who is tired and overwrought. He might well begin to have paranoia and confusion over who is friend and who is foe. The immune system can be compared to this soldier, as it is the guardian of the individuals' body against infectious agents and dangerous substances.

Sometimes free-floating stuff can create fatigue and weakness. These unpleasant symptoms occur because the various parts of the body where the stuff may settle for a period can find it difficult to function with the stuff sitting in them. An individual may experience fatigue in any body part with no obvious cause. He or she may feel weak in any area, again with no visible reason. Continuing to use a muscle that feels weak can make that muscle tired and fatigued. These symptoms are difficult to diagnose, uncomfortable and they can be frightening since nobody can give a definite diagnosis.

As the free-floating stuff moves around in the body, it can affect the person's emotional equilibrium as well. Often individuals will report the experience of a feeling of "something is not quite right" though it is difficult for them to describe adequately. These rather unclear symptoms are enough to make the individual feel anxious. They sometimes describe feelings of dread along with the anxiety, as if something unpleasant is going to happen although they cannot explain what it might be.

Many mental health diagnoses are also related to free-floating stuff, because the vague feelings of dread or anxiety are most often treated by mental health professionals. Since each individual will react to the feelings in different ways, any number of diagnoses can be appropriate. This is especially true when there are no physical manifestations of the stuff.

While any number of mental health diagnoses can be appropriate depending on how the individual reacts to the feelings of dread and anxiety, some are fairly common. These include the various anxiety disorders, phobias, and panic disorders. The vague feelings of anxiety and dread can cause behaviors that seem to demonstrate excessive fear and unreasonable anxiety. Some individuals develop panic disorders because of very strong fear of feeling the anxiety.

As we discussed in the section on Replay Stuff, these disorders can cause behaviors that are unsettling for the individual as well as those around him or her. These behaviors can cause social stigmatization, which can cause more stress and unhappiness, which causes more anxiety and so on.

How Do I Determine If I Have Free-Floating Stuff

This checklist was designed to assist individuals as they learn about and work with Free-Floating Stuff. Please use it to help you find out whether this type of stuff is an issue for you. Again, please remember that it is a starting point.

1. Do I tire more easily than other people? Y/N

2. Do I seem to catch every "bug" that is going around? Y/N

3. Do I have sensitivities or allergies to many things? Y/N

4. Have I been diagnosed with an autoimmune disorder? Y/N

5. Do I feel a sense of dread? Y/N

6. Do I have anxious feelings without obvious cause? Y/N

7. Have I got a diagnosed or obvious anxiety disorder? Y/N

8. Do others tell me to "relax" frequently? Y/N

9. Do I worry about my health whether or not I visit doctors often? Y/N

10. Does my anxious behavior cause me social problems? Y/N

If you answered "yes" to any question, you might be experiencing free-floating stuff. The more "yes" answers you gave, the more likely it is that you are dealing with this type of stuff. You can use this information as a starting point for addressing, loosening, and removing this stuff.

Anyone experiencing situations that appear to relate to free-floating stuff can do a number of things. First, go ahead and treat the symptoms as you see fit. Good things to do for the fatigue and anxiety would include massage and relaxation through whatever type of meditation, yoga, or other practice suits the individual. For the anxiety, talk therapy can be wonderful if the individual benefits from understanding how their behavior affects others or can learn ways to manage their anxiety. Anti-anxiety medications can be useful when used judiciously in conjunction with other forms of therapy. For autoimmune disorders and weakness, a good healthy diet and regular exercise as appropriate will help to strengthen the body and encourage the stuff to begin to loosen. Following the Simple **Steps to Wellness** listed later in this book is essential when dealing with these types of situations.

Other modalities such as acupuncture, Reiki, reflexology and so on may serve to increase the feeling of well-being and increase the energy available to function. Appropriate counseling or even medications may be needed to reduce the feelings of dread and anxiety to manageable levels. Hypnosis and EFT could also be used effectively in this situation. These things are important so the individual has the energy and strength to work to remove the stuff permanently. You can read about these and other techniques in the **Loosening Techniques** section of this book.

A person who is experiencing the effects of free-floating stuff is not weak or subject to blame. All people have, at some time or another, had enough free-floating stuff in their systems to produce an effect. These effects can be fleeting, like a cold or a moment of anxiousness for "no reason" or they can become chronic and develop into a long-term illness. Individuals who get frequent colds, who suffer from changing food or environmental sensitivities or who seem to develop infections every time they get a scratch may have a problem with free-floating stuff. Regardless, the effects of free-floating stuff, like those of the other types of stuff, can and will generally get better or go away when the stuff is removed.

Loosening Techniques

There are some wonderful techniques for loosening stuff, some of which have already been mentioned. The most qualified practitioner you can find should provide these techniques. Individuals should NOT read these descriptions and attempt to work on themselves or their families. However, a basic understanding of some of these techniques will help you to find the practitioners and techniques best suited to your situation. For practitioners in your area, please check a good resource guide such as the **Whole Life Pages,** the services directory at the end of this book or resources in your own community.

The Emotional Freedom Technique (EFT) is excellent for loosening all three types of stuff. This technique, while seemingly simple, should be provided and taught by a qualified therapist. The most likely type of therapist who would offer EFT would be a hypnotherapist. The basic theory behind EFT is that emotions are created and stored in the electrical system of the body. By tapping on specific spots, similar to acupuncture points, an electrical circuit is created. These spots are on the acupuncture meridians, which relate to the major organs and systems of the body. Specific phrases are spoken and repeated as these points are tapped in a prescribed order. With each "round" of

EFT, the troubling emotions recede and are never felt in the same way again. EFT is simple and easy enough that the average person can be trained to use it at home for his or her own work. It is important, however, to work with a qualified therapist to ensure that you are using the technique correctly for yourself, and laypeople should never, ever work on others. EFT is intended to be quick, inexpensive, and functional. Most therapists who do EFT with their clients will work with the person for one or two sessions and teach the individual to work on their own after that. It is rare indeed for anyone to require multiple sessions costing a significant amount of money.

Time Line Therapy™ is excellent for reducing the hold that an emotion or situation has on the individual. It is a content-free technique that is used by hypnotherapists when working with people whose stuff keeps them in a stuck place or has created significant difficulties. Emotions are addressed, but not specific memories. Because it is free of content, the individual does not need to know or remember the specific events or emotions that caused the stuff in the first place. This means that there is no risk of increasing the critical mass of the stuff. In addition, the individual need not experience the uncomfortable situations again. It is most useful when dealing with critical mass stuff, though it can be effective in loosening some unconscious replay stuff as well. While free-floating stuff is smaller than the other two types, it can be addressed using Time Line Therapy if the emotions can be identified. As there are no side effects to consider, it can be attempted in any of these situations in complete safety. Again, a qualified hypnotherapist is the appropriate professional to work with in this way.

Hypnotherapy is the use of hypnosis for therapeutic reasons. A qualified hypnotherapist is a graduate of a training program that is approved by at least one of the major hypnosis organizations. As there is no state certification or licensure in any state at the time of this writing (2004) the reputable organizations listed in the back of this book are some of the public's best means of ensuring proper training for a hypnotherapist. Some psychologists and psychiatrists, as well as other professionals, may receive training in hypnosis as a part of their professional education. The quality and amount of this training varies widely, so if you choose to work with your other practitioner in hypnosis it is a good idea to ask about their hypnosis training and experience. Hypnosis is a state of deep relaxation in which the individual is more able to follow suggestions that lead to what he or she wants and is more in contact with his or her unconscious mind. It is safe, effective, and comfortable. There are no "side effects" or dangers inherent in hypnotherapy and no harm can result from properly induced hypnosis. However, if the practitioner is not well trained, you may not receive the services you need to loosen your stuff. Most of the major hypnotherapy organizations maintain referral lists and would be able to help find a qualified practitioner in most places.

Talk Therapies are those processes generally referred to as counseling or psychotherapy. Psychologists, licensed clinical social workers, pastoral counselors, and psychiatrists usually offer talk therapies. These can include individual and group therapy sessions and take place over time. Talk therapy is very familiar to most Americans from depictions of these modalities in movies and television. Talk therapy is most effective in loosening both the critical mass stuff and the replay stuff that is available to the conscious mind. It can also be useful in addressing the emotional and behavioral effects of free-floating stuff and replay stuff as well. That is because talk therapy works with the conscious mind and its understanding of the situation. Often with these types of stuff a conscious understanding makes it easier to let the stuff go. Therefore, while talk therapy is not generally effective in removing stuff, it is often essential in loosening its hold so that removal is possible. Licensure and other requirements generally vary from state to state in the United States and from country to country in Europe and other places. In most places, referrals are available from the licensing bodies or professional organizations to which the therapists may belong.

Cognitive-Behavioral Therapy utilizes the individual's understanding and behavioral changes to loosen the stuff. This is very helpful when specific behaviors tend to allow the stuff to gather or to reinforce its effects. A qualified therapist, usually a psychologist, would be the appropriate professional to work with in this way. Sometimes called "behavior modification" this therapy works to address any behavioral component of the individual's condition. It is important to note that not all medical conditions have a behavioral cause or even a behavioral component. One area in which Cognitive-Behavioral Therapy is extremely useful is in situations in which the individual has learned to control others or their environment by using their condition. Sometimes these individuals can be very manipulative, which makes it harder for those assisting them to remove their stuff. Sometimes it can be difficult for them to give up their condition as it provides them with hidden benefits in so many ways. If the individual is willing, they can be taught new ways to get what they need without resorting to manipulation or needing to hold onto their stuff. This sort of therapy can be very useful in addressing the anxious behaviors that replay or free-floating stuff can cause and which can result in social stigmatization. Congnitive-Behavioral Therapy is often depicted as a system of rewards and punishments, which is not really accurate. While rewards are inherent in the treatment as the person learns to meet these needs more appropriately, punishments are inappropriate. The natural consequence of not having the need met in the old way is appropriate and it is not a punishment. Cognitive-Behavioral Therapy is most effective when working with replay stuff that is close enough to the conscious mind and in addressing some behavioral effects of all types of stuff. The American Association of Behavioral Therapists maintains a referral network of therapists in America who are trained and well qualified in this modality. Their information is available in the Resource Directory located at the end of this book.

Massage Therapy is excellent for loosening up the body and reminding the individual how it feels to have less pain and looser muscles. It is wonderful for addressing the physical effects of all three major types of stuff. A good, qualified massage therapist can work with the individual to relax the body and reduce the effects of the stuff, as well as often helping the person to avoid allowing the stuff to gather again. Massage drains the lymphatic system, removes lactic acid, and increases the body's endorphins. Lactic acid is the waste product from muscle use and damage, and it causes significant pain when left in the muscles. Endorphins are hormones that have been described as the body's opiate equivalent, being 700 times stronger than morphine. In specific conditions, massage can make a dramatic difference, even reducing pain and increasing motivation to get well. However, lymphomas and some other illnesses are considered contraindications for massage therapy. A qualified massage therapist will be able to advise you. Massage therapy feels good, but it should never be sexual in any way. Your body should be draped and covered with sheets at all times, with only the area being worked exposed carefully. Massage therapy is regulated and licensure is available in many states. The two major massage therapy organizations listed in the Resource Directory at the end of this book will be able to help you find a qualified therapist in your area who is in compliance with all regulations governing the practice of massage.

Cranio-Sacral Therapy is excellent for addressing many of the issues arising from Critical Mass stuff which may sit in the fluid of the spine. The therapeutic technique is used by specially trained practitioners, typically physical therapists, massage therapists and chiropractors. The aim of the technique is to allow for the free flow of the fluid, as it was intended to flow. Practitioners are trained by the Upledger Institute, which maintains all credentialing and offers a referral service.

Visceral Manipulation is another therapy taught by the Upledger Institute, whose information is available in the Resource List at the end of this book. This gentle yet effective technique is utilized by trained practitioners, usually physical therapists and massage therapists, to assist in reestablishing the flow and function of the intestinal area. This therapeutic technique is beneficial in relieving the discomfort experienced by people whose stuff has settled in their digestive tracts and caused symptoms such as diarrhea, gas, constipation and intestinal pain.

Reiki is an ancient healing art from Japan. The theory behind Reiki is clear and simple. Reiki is a form of energy work that works to remove blockages that are constricting the flow of energy in the body. Reiki clears the **Chakras,** which are described as energy vortexes within the body that allow the energy to flow as it should through the physical body. These vortexes are in the form of wheels. The word *Chakra* means *Wheel.* When the blockages are gone and the Chakras are clear, the individual experiences increased energy and health. For centuries, individual clients have described these experiences as a result of Reiki treatment sessions. Reiki is done with the client lying on a table or other surface, fully clothed apart from the shoes. The practitioner will place the hands above the body or rest them lightly on the body while the energy is balanced. Universal energy is brought in to create and maintain that balance. Much about Reiki is mysterious, such as the secret symbols the practitioner may utilize, but it has become quite mainstream and accepted in American life. Often, massage therapists, hypnotherapists and other alternative health workers are also Reiki practitioners, though Reiki stands alone.

Acupuncture is an ancient Chinese healing modality that utilizes the meridians, or energy pathways in the body to balance **chi** or life force energy. Energy can be increased or lessened in a specific location, according to what the individual needs. Millions of individual clients over hundreds of years have experienced benefits from acupuncture, and the use of specific points for specific complaints has been well documented. Practitioners are trained using this information. The training requires copying and memorization of this information as well as point location and needle usage skills. Individuals report increases in feelings of well-being, relief from pain and better overall health. Acupuncture is most useful when dealing with energy-draining effects of critical mass stuff and replay stuff. It can also be used very effectively to move free-floating stuff to another location or even loosening it to the point that it leaves the body. Thin, solid needles are used and placed in specific locations along the meridians. Most reports indicate that a skilled acupuncturist can insert the needles with little discomfort to the patient. Acupuncture should therefore be performed only by a well-qualified acupuncturist with many hundreds of hours of training. In most states, there is regulation and licensure for acupuncturists, though in some states other practitioners such as chiropractors are allowed to train for shorter durations and offer acupuncture as an adjunct to their regular practice.

Acupressure is similar to acupuncture although there is one major difference. In acupressure, there are no needles. The practitioner uses finger pressure on the same points as in acupuncture. Often the results are similar to acupuncture. It can be used in situations where the individual may be uncomfortable with needles, or where there are other considerations that would indicate that needles ought not to be used. Generally, acupressure is offered by acupuncturists because the training and information is the same, apart from the use of needles and actually puncturing the skin. There is no licensure available for acupressure.

Process Acupressure is a form of acupressure that includes emotional release work. The therapist presses on various parts of the body and holds gentle pressure while addressing the emotions that come up. This is great for replay stuff particularly, though some individuals find relief from critical mass stuff as well, if the emotion that is at the core of the stuff is found and addressed. The emotional basis of free-floating stuff can be addressed in this way as well, though there might not be enough of these emotions for the individual to find and release them during a treatment. If the individual has several treatments, it is more likely that the "smaller" emotions will surface. This modality is generally used by acupuncturists and massage therapists who have additional training. Persons entering into this type of therapy needs to make sure the therapist is someone with whom they can feel comfortable letting down their guard. Process acupressure does not require a license and there are no licenses available for practitioners of this technique.

Zero Balancing is another modality that works with the body and emotions. In Zero Balancing, the client is fully clothed on a massage table and the practitioner applies gentle traction and/or pressure to parts of the body. The result is a feeling of looseness, comfort, and relaxation. For individuals who are feeling a lot of tightness or stiffness, this modality is very pleasant. Because they feel more loose and comfortable, they may remember how it feels to feel good. They may well loosen the stuff significantly as a result of the new looseness and comfort of their body. Zero Balancing is beneficial in all types of stuff, though it seems to address the issues arising from free-floating stuff particularly well. Practitioners are often massage therapists or other bodyworkers. There is no licensure available for these practitioners.

Shiatsu is an ancient form of bodywork from Japan. It uses pressure as well as stretching. Shiatsu is usually done on a mat on the floor, though a massage table can be used if it is more comfortable for the client. Unlike massage therapy, Shiatsu does not require the removal of clothing other than shoes. Like Zero Balancing, Shiatsu leaves the individual with a feeling of physical well-being that can easily translate to the loosening of the stuff that has made them less than well. Often this motivates the individual to work toward removal of the stuff permanently. This modality is excellent for loosening free-floating stuff, as it is a whole body modality so it can address the small bits of stuff throughout the body. A well-trained practitioner can assist the individual to reduce or loosen the free-floating stuff while relaxing the body and addressing the results of the stuff.

Ayurveda is a system of health care from India. The basic theory behind Ayurveda is that there are three main body types, which relate to shape, energy, and other factors. Individuals are thought to have differing needs depending upon their body type. Using information about the individual's body type and other particulars, as well as what they are experiencing in their health, the practitioner makes nutritional and other lifestyle recommendations. Balance is a goal of Ayurvedic practice. The recommendations made by the practitioner are intended to lead to balance and better health. Critical mass stuff-induced illness and disease can often be improved with this modality to the point that the individual is able to begin to reduce and remove their stuff. A new feeling of health can often be very motivating. A well-trained Ayurvedic practitioner would be able to offer these recommendations as well as other treatments as appropriate. Ayurveda is effective in loosening all three types of stuff, because there are so many aspects of life that are addressed in this system of healthcare.

Nutrition is very important for everyone. However, when you are loosening and removing stuff, it is vital that the body be as well nourished as possible. There are a number of opinions about what proper nutrition is, and enough books and systems of attaining good nutritional health to fill a warehouse. Probably the most sensible way of going about this is to find a qualified dietician or nutritionist whom you trust and ask questions about these issues. Ask your body if the suggestions are appropriate and acceptable. You will find information on how to communicate with your body later in this book. However, if you ask your body a question and notice a happy feeling then the answer is "yes" and if you get an uncomfortable feeling then it is not. Only if the suggestions are appropriate for your body should you consider following them. Remember, no one system is appropriate for everyone and your body will tell you what it needs to eat to be healthy if you will only ask it. Regardless of the type or types of stuff you are addressing, a good nutritional status is necessary if you are to be successful in reducing and removing your stuff. Nutritionists are licensed in many jurisdictions. You can also find a qualified nutritionist by contacting one of the organizations listed in the Resource Directory at the end of this book.

Chiropractic Care is offered by trained, licensed Doctors of Chiropractic. By manipulating the spine and other parts of the body, a chiropractor seeks to relieve dysfunction, pain, and misalignments (called subluxations) from the body. This is again useful in loosening the stuff, especially critical mass stuff and free-floating stuff, that causes physical ailments while addressing some of the symptoms the individual may be experiencing. Often beginning to feel better is the catalyst that causes the individual to seek to remove the stuff permanently. Good chiropractic care is a part of maintaining general good health and preventing stuff from accumulating once it has been removed or at least loosened. A regular schedule of chiropractic care is useful in removing pain, increasing endorphins and maintaining healthy function while actually allowing the body to become stronger so that the removal of stuff is easier and more comfortable. Chiropractors are licensed in most jurisdictions. You can find a qualified chiropractor in your area by checking the Resource Directory in this book, contacting your local Chamber of Commerce or asking your friends and relatives which chiropractors they prefer. You will be surprised how many of the people you know visit a chiropractor regularly!

Western Medicine has a significant place in loosening stuff. Very often, proponents of natural healing will forget this, and some will even deny it, but it is true. Often critical mass stuff has accumulated in one area of the body to such a degree that a physical growth or other dysfunctional situation has developed that must be surgically removed or treated with medicines to allow the person to survive. Frequently, the stuff has caused a situation in which medication is required for the body to function while carrying that stuff. At other times, the results of stuff can be so unpleasant that medication is required to alleviate the discomfort, both physical and mental. This is reasonable and valid. It is not the only way to address the results of stuff-created problems, but it is often at least a temporary part of the solution to those problems and the discomfort they cause. With the appropriate use of Western medicine, the individual can be more comfortable and ready to work on loosening all three types of stuff. It is a very good idea to find a Western medical practitioner who understands your situation and how you wish to address it. Most doctors are reasonable human beings who understand that the individual dealing with the stuff-caused condition is, in fact, the real expert on that condition as it manifests in his or her body. The individual is also the only one who knows how it feels to live with the health condition and what he or she want to do about it. By choosing and even interviewing doctors, it is possible for any individual to find the best helper for the particular situation which that body is experiencing at that time. There are many directories of physicians and hospitals available in almost every area. These often include philosophical or mission statements from the individual physicians, which can be used to help individuals to choose the most appropriate practitioner for their own needs and situation. The practice of Western Medicine is regulated and licensed in every jurisdiction.

A Word About Adaptive Equipment: Adaptive Equipment is any object that people use to accomplish any of the Activities of Daily Living (known to doctors and therapists as ADLs) that their medical condition would seem to preclude. This includes such things as wheelchairs for those who cannot walk or who cannot walk distances, reacher/grabbers, magnifying glasses and so on. Using these things when needed is not an admission of defeat or a sign of weakness. It is the most logical thing to do under the circumstances, period. We seem to understand that this is so in the case of glasses for those who need assistance with their vision, but not with other disabling conditions. It is a sign of common sense in a difficult situation and it is an affirmation of life.

I used a wheelchair for ten years, give or take a couple of months. It allowed me to shop with my daughter for all of her prom dresses, go on family vacations, go to parents' nights at the schools my children attended and to pursue my career. Without my wheelchair, I would have been unable to do much of anything; I would have been relegated to my home and bored to tears. I would never have gotten well because I would not have known it was possible and I would probably been afraid or unable to venture out to find out about the possibilities. The point of this story is to absolutely insist that those who use adaptive equipment are in life, not hiding from it. They are working toward having the most normal life possible for them at that moment and should be treated and honored as such.

Adaptive devices can and should be used with joy and a sense of fun. I felt a bit awkward when I began to use a scooter-style wheelchair, I will admit. I met someone one day who told me that I had the best toys, and I chose to see my devices in that light. After that, I had a lot of fun taking my young niece up and down the stairs on my Stair-glider or letting her ride on the scooter with me. I did enjoy the little kids asking why I got to ride my bike in the mall and they could not. One dear child told me that I used a cane because I was "very old" and I had to agree. I am quite sure that 41 looked positively ancient from the vantage point of three! If someone in your life uses adaptive devices with less than happiness or resists using what would make their life more livable, play with it. Make up silly songs or activities around the device. Be really creative. If you have been resisting any equipment that would make your life easier or more fun, even temporarily while you get rid of the stuff that created your current situation, get that equipment! Use it with gratitude and fun and, when you are done needing it, pass it on!

Primary Gains

There are sometimes legitimate gains that people receive as a result of a stuff-generated condition. After all, we gain from any experience we have in life. It is said that our experiences shape our personalities. This is true because we learn skills as we adapt to whatever situation we are in, whether it is perceived as negative or positive. Our appropriate coping mechanisms can become our strengths.

There is no need to lose the legitimate gains, sometimes called **primary gains** that come to any individual as a result of learning to live with a stuff-caused condition. I certainly received a lot of primary gains as a result of my former disability of muscular dystrophy. I learned to trust my own perceptions, ask for what I need, respect my body and most importantly that I am me regardless of immediate situation. I have been told that I dealt with the disability with grace and humor, if that is true I am grateful for those skills and glad that I will have them to draw on regardless of what events occur in my life in the future.

Primary gains are wonderful gifts we receive when we are dealing with a "problem" situation. We gave them to ourselves as we were dealing with the situation since they are the things we learned and the skills we developed for ourselves. We get to keep them when we get well. We can use these skills and attributes in any way we desire. One interesting fact is that, as we are no longer dealing with the results of the stuff, we can use the skills and attributes we gained in new and more creative ways. Our energy is no longer focused on dealing with the stuff so we can invest that energy in new endeavors, using whatever we gained as we addressed our stuff, but in new and more interesting ways.

I have a dear friend who experiences some of the mental health challenges that can result from replay or free-floating stuff. As my friend has gone through her life with this experience, she has learned wonderful coping mechanisms. These include thinking "outside the box" as well as humor, analytical thinking and even gentleness. She is brilliant and believes that some of her brilliance is a result of needing to use her intelligence to work out the things that she did not understand due to her challenges. My friend's humor is the stuff of legend; she is a truly funny person when she chooses to express herself in that way. Her analytical abilities have been honed by her having to figure out the behavior of others and her own reactions. Because my friend feels unhappy when others are not gentle and kind toward her, she is careful to speak kindly and to treat others gently. She understands that she can get well, totally remove her stuff, and retain the skills she has gained.

My friend can use her brilliance, ability to see things in different ways, gentleness and humor in any way she wants once she is no longer using these attributes for survival. I can use my respect for my perceptions and my alleged humor as I write, teach, and work with my clients, as well as in my family life. We can both delight in the things we discover we can do.

Secondary Gains

For many people, there are inappropriate or unhealthy benefits to having their stuff or the results of their stuff. Until and unless these benefits are addressed it will be difficult if not impossible for these individuals to release their stuff. The clinical term for these benefits is **secondary gains.**

Secondary gains can be anything and everything a person receives, usually from others, because of any situation in life. These situations are usually "unfortunate" ones, such as disabilities, medical conditions, and economic or other problems. The secondary gains are the silver linings in the clouds cast by the situation. However, unlike primary gains, secondary gains are neither helpful nor appropriate in any long-term way. Secondary gains are not the same as new skills or attributes an individual can take into other situations and use well. They are generally things the individual gains that are only available if they continue being ill or having their stuff.

Do not underestimate the importance of secondary gains. They are sometimes called the glue that keeps people stuck in old patterns, behaviors and beliefs that no longer serve them. After a time, the individual may come to expect and even rely on these gains. They often experience fear or discomfort when they think about living without these things. They may not like to think about being "one of the crowd" as they negotiate their day. They may have forgotten how to do it without the gains.

Secondary gains can be the things society does to make a more level playing field for disabled people, such as special entrances to the roller coaster. They can be the way some people are kind and allow the individual to get in front of them in line at the grocery store or assist them in reaching items. They can be the extra attention from friends and loved ones or the way individuals are often catered to in social or work situations. They can be things most of us would not want, which become important to the individual, such as relationships with and attention from care providers and even "disability" or "condition" charities and groups. Truly, secondary gains can be and are anything the person perceives as desirable that they can only have if they remain disabled or ill.

Because I had muscular dystrophy and needed to use a wheelchair, I got put at the front of lines in amusement parks, got the best parking spots, and was noticed more easily in public places. This often resulted in special experiences that I did enjoy. Some of the time, I needed the assistance that I received in order to accomplish the things I wanted to do. Now I can do those things without any assistance at all. It can seem to be easier to have others do things, but it is not. I personally prefer doing things my way when I want to do them. It can be frustrating to have to wait until others are able to assist with tasks or to have to accept that some things will be done differently from how I would do them.

In order to receive help and the interesting experiences I got as a disabled person, I had to retain my disability. When I got well, I found that I did not have the pain and weakness from the muscular dystrophy but I had to do things for myself. I needed to get to the point where I preferred the daily experience of wellness and independence to the "goodies" I was getting. At that point, I was able to let go of my stuff and get well.

Until and unless people get to the point where they can honestly say that they are willing and able to let go of the secondary gains they are receiving because of their stuff-induced conditions, they will find it difficult if not impossible to release their stuff. They may be able to loosen it temporarily, but it will remain. They may even get relief from a medical condition, but if the stuff is still there, it will reappear either in the same way if it is replay or critical mass stuff or in a very different way if it is free-floating stuff. We often see this happen when people appear to get over a serious medical condition only to develop something else pretty quickly. This happens when the individual successfully gets rid of enough stuff to become healthy but misses the secondary gains so much that he or she unconsciously manufactures enough stuff to receive them again.

It is very important that we understand that this manufacture of another (or the same) condition is an unconscious behavior. No blame attaches to it; it is absolutely not something the individual consciously chooses to do. In fact, they may consciously feel very upset and angry that another challenge has come their way, not understanding how this happened. In order to help the individual avoid this pitfall, friends and family members need to be sure that their loved one is made aware of the good things that are happening now that the stuff and its related problems are gone.

While the individual must be the one to decide when it is appropriate to get rid of his or her stuff, friends can lovingly point out the secondary gains they observe. However, this needs to be done gently and respectfully. Family and friends must be clear in their own minds that it is the individual's life and not theirs so they can point it out once or twice but never nag. In fact, after mentioning that there is a secondary gain situation it should be left alone unless the individual asks for help. People do not usually like to be told that they are receiving secondary gains; it sounds like criticism or blame. Friends and family must be very careful to avoid even the appearance of anything like that. Any harping on the subject is likely to have the opposite effect; the person will ignore the friends or relatives who are legitimately trying to help. This is not stubbornness or foolishly childish behavior. It is the legitimate response of someone who is being pushed to deal with things before he or she is ready.

Friends and family members of someone who is dealing with a stuff-related condition have a choice. They are quite free to stop offering the type of assistance or service that they perceive as unhealthy for themselves. They can discuss with the individual what their own needs are and how they intend to meet them. Lovingly assuring the individual that they are not abandoning him or her, just that they need to take care of their own health and well-being (otherwise they will begin to feel resentful and may develop a stuff-related condition of their own) they can take back some of their own power and make sure they stay well. They can also discuss how to meet everyone's needs. What they should never do is beg, whine, or plead to be let out of a task. If everyone is an adult about this sort of situation, it will generally resolve quite readily.

It can be difficult to determine when there are secondary gains, but there are often clues that we can use to determine that we or those we love are obtaining secondary gains from a situation. Some of the things that point out obvious secondary gain situations include remarks the individual makes. These are called *verbal pointers* to the secondary gain. If your friend says, "I'm not well" in a gleeful tone or as a reason why you need to accommodate some outlandish request, this is a good clue that we are dealing with a verbal pointer. If the individual becomes annoyed when asked to do things or make accommodations for others, using the idea that "I'm not well" as the reason for this annoyance, there is a sure verbal pointer to a secondary gain. Obviously, the secondary gain is getting one's own way all the time!

Another common verbal pointer is a statement of how "naughty" the individual was in some way. For example, a young woman with a disability was unable to feel anything below the waist, and as a result had managed to get a fairly severe burn on her buttocks. She was unable to feel the burn or its treatment, yet she yelled and fought the nurses who were attempting to help her to heal and avoid infection. There was no logical reason for her to behave in this fashion; the treatment was not causing her any discomfort after all. However, she got a great deal of pleasure in telling the other patients in the burn unit that she had hit the nurse. She was clearly deriving a secondary gain from this situation.

Sometimes the individual delightedly remarks on what he or she has managed to get from others inappropriately. Maybe someone kindly offers additional products or services to a person who appears to them to be disabled or ill. This is kind but if the person gets used to it, it becomes a secondary gain he or she comes to expect and even manipulate situations to obtain. It pays to be especially vigilant about this behavior, because it shows that there is a huge secondary gain that may tend to get in the way of removing the stuff. Individuals can gently and politely refuse the offers of extra goods and services, because they are very kindly meant but unhealthy for the recipient.

One other verbal pointer you are likely to encounter is a comment on what the individual cannot do. While this may occur on occasion in context with anyone with a challenge, if it happens frequently or out of context, it is a verbal pointer. For example, it is appropriate for a person who cannot walk to mention that he or she cannot enter a specific inaccessible restaurant and suggest a different place for dinner. It is a verbal pointer when the person who cannot walk mentions it in situations where it is not an issue or where the other person obviously understands that the individual cannot walk.

If the disability inappropriately becomes the main topic of conversation, the verbal pointer may itself be a secondary gain. In this situation, the individual becomes the center of attention in the social situation. Friends and relatives are almost afraid to ask, "How are you?" because of the long, involved and complaining answer they will receive.

In addition to verbal pointers, there are other clues to secondary gains. If there is some obvious gain that most people would find reinforcing, then it is likely that there is secondary gain. One area where this occurs for women more than men is in the care taking of the spouse or other significant person in the individual's life. Women are the caretakers in most relationships, but when a woman's stuff-induced condition prevents her from doing things for her family or herself, the other adults in her life take over. For the first time since childhood, in some cases, others are preparing meals, doing laundry or other tasks in order to help the woman who is unable to cope as she used to do. Naturally, this relief from work when she is truly not feeling her best is wonderful. Those who take over tasks are doing the right and appropriate thing. If they are capable of doing some of the household chores, the rest of the family ought to be doing so anyway. However, this secondary gain may be stronger than her desire to be well. A man may experience the same sort of secondary gain if his chores and onerous tasks are taken over by others when he is not able to do them. Children who are not required to go to school or do homework or household chores as their siblings must can also experience it.

Some secondary gains are harder for the non-affected friends and relatives to understand. This is because that which is gained does not seem to be something anyone would want.

In some cases, the relationships the person develops with healthcare providers, both conventional and alternative, can be significant. It is easier to understand if we realize that some individuals have worked with the same providers for several years and have developed a level of comfort or security with those people. The providers are there to do a job and may not be able to continue to see someone who is well. They may not believe that wellness is possible when dealing with whatever the particular condition might be. It may be just a bit uncomfortable for the providers to have to think outside of that particular box. At any rate, healthy people are unlikely to continue to need to see their providers on a regular basis.

If the individual has joined a "condition-based" organization or social group then there may well be important relationships there as well. The unspoken fear is likely to be that if the person gets well they will have to sever these relationships. Sometimes, getting well is seen as a betrayal by others who are continuing to deal with the medical condition. It is almost as if those "left behind" are feeling that the world will expect them to get well when they are not ready or believe it cannot be done, which creates a great deal of fear which can turn to anger with the well person. This anger is unnecessary and will be easily dealt with as long as the newly well person makes it clear that he or she does not think any less of friends who are still dealing with the condition.

Spending time with medical people or in situations where most of the people have a specific medical condition would not appeal to many people. However, for some individuals whose stuff has caused their world to shrink to such a degree that these interactions are meaningful in the scope of their lives, they are vital links to the world of people and activity. If most friends are not available due to differences in schedule or ability, medical personnel can become significant relationships. People who do not have social outlets due to their stuff-induced medical conditions often join disease-related organizations in order to have activities and interactions that are planned and organized in ways that do not challenge them physically. This is a sad but true secondary gain. The loss of these relationships and activities can be devastating if they are not replaced with more healthy ones.

Am I Receiving Secondary Gains from My Stuff?

Please answer these questions honestly. You do not need to show your answer to anyone. This self-quiz is intended to allow individuals to determine if there any secondary gains that may be in the way of their getting rid of their stuff.

1. Are people nicer to me now that I have a challenge? Y/N

2. Are my family and friends more helpful to me now? Y/N

3. Do people I do not know offer to assist me? Y/N

4. Do I get better services than other, well, people? Y/N

5. Do I get my own way in social situations more often than not? Y/N

6. Do I look forward to seeing my care providers for non-medical reasons? Y/N

7. Are my relationships with these providers important to me? Y/N

8. Do I belong to any "condition-related" organizations? Y/N
9. Are my relationships within the organization important to me? Y/N
10. Do I fear the loss of any of these relationships? Y/N

If you answered "yes" to any questions, you may be dealing with some secondary gain. The more "yes" answers you had, the more likely this is to be the case. It is up to you to decide whether you wish to address this situation which might be impeding your ability to remove your stuff and get well.

Neutralizing Secondary Gains

Secondary gains exist. There is little point in denying this fact. Most situations create secondary gains if they are to be maintained. It is important, therefore, to neutralize these secondary gains. To neutralize a secondary gain means to render it impotent, to make sure it has no power any more. To do this we need to analyze the gain to determine what need it meets for the individual and find a more appropriate and healthy way to meet this need.

Stuff-generated conditions and disabilities create situations. These situations give rise to secondary gains that in various ways meet needs the individual has. Each individual will create ways to meet the needs that are specific to him or her, whatever those exact needs and desires might be. The ways these needs are met will vary widely from person to person based on the needs as he or she experiences and perceive them, and the ways in which he or she would like them to be met.

We discussed the woman whose physical condition prevented her from doing heavy housework, carrying laundry, and so on. Her husband and children took over these tasks when she developed a disabling condition so that she could conserve her energy and strength for working at her highly paid executive job and doing some of the other tasks of her life. Before her illness, she had done all of the laundry and other household chores while her husband and nearly-grown children did little or nothing around the house. Her resentment, along with other situations in her childhood and adult life, combined to create critical mass stuff, which resulted in a muscle disorder. In order to release this stuff, she and her family had to come to an agreement on meeting her reasonable need to not do all the work. This agreement was predicated on the idea that she could be well and still have other people do their fair share of the physical drudgery work at home. She was then free to release the stuff and regain her health without fear of returning to what had been a very unfair division of labor. This is a situation in which the secondary gain was obvious and other family members were willing and able to cooperate without any difficulty.

Sometimes, secondary gains are harder to recognize and address. If, for example, the individual has become accustomed to receiving "special" treatment in daily life due to a stuff-related condition, it may be harder to identify and address these gains. Society is not about to continue to offer "handicapped" parking, seating, and other benefits to healthy people, nor should we expect that. These things are intended to create a "level playing field" so that individuals with disabilities can function more effectively alongside others without disabilities.

It is very easy to develop a sense of entitlement, and it is understandable that it does develop. If someone is being offered special privileges every day for a number of years, and if those offering these privileges are offended when they are not wanted, an individual begins to accept them, then to expect them and finally to demand them at times. Dealing with this type of secondary gain is not as simple as getting the rest of the family to do their chores.

So, how do we address this entitled feeling that some people develop? If we are not the individuals who have developed the sense of entitlement, there is really very little we can do. The only thing we can do is to refuse to participate. If a friend or relative begins to act entitled to our time, possessions, or efforts we can choose whether to give them what they are demanding or not. If we choose not to participate, we would do well to explain our reasons and stand firm on what we are willing to do. We can expect some anger and resentment from our friend or relative, but we need to do what is most appropriate for us. Their needs can be met in a different, healthier way.

If you have a stuff-generated medical condition and your friends and relatives are doing things for you, you might come to expect that they will continue indefinitely and even do more as time goes on. While they may be willing at first, if you are not grateful, polite, and reasonable with them, they will probably find it difficult to continue. In short, if you behave as if you feel entitled to their time, money, or efforts, or if you actually begin to feel that you are entitled, you can expect that others will eventually feel unappreciated and overburdened. In time, they will not be able to continue because it would be unhealthy for them. When your friends and relatives tell you that they are going to have to stop assisting you in the same way or that the relationship has become one-way, listen and do your best to understand what they are telling you. You might feel fear because you rely on them, but please do not react with anger or resentment. Remember that your needs can be met in another way.

Special treatment sets a person apart from others. Most people see this as innocuous and fair; and, to be perfectly honest, special assistance is sometimes necessary. It is also true that individuals who offer special treatment are usually trying to be nice and kind to someone they see as needing help. While special treatment or extra help is sometimes needed, it occasionally makes the regular activities of life more convenient for individuals needing assistance than for the rest of the community. The idea is to make life equal, not better for one group than for another. If life is more convenient when a person's stuff-caused condition creates a disability, then that convenience is a secondary gain that must be neutralized.

In order to neutralize this type of gain, the individual must choose to be healthy in all ways. The individual must determine that these "goodies" are not worth the cost of having health issues or a disability. In order to remove the stuff that causes the condition, the individual must be prepared to neutralize this gain. As people begin to heal, they must begin to remove these "treats" from their lives and replace them with other ways of being special. While this will vary from person to person, of course, many people have found that doing something that sets them apart in a desirable way can really offset the loss of special privileges. Some individuals have even become athletes in an effort to develop a positive recognition factor for their own specialness. Others have chosen to develop their talents in artistic or professional areas or simply to volunteer in their communities in ways that got them positive recognition from others.

Recognition for a positive attribute or behavior feels much better than the pity-tinged recognition they may have experienced before. Often the only disabled member of a church congregation, for example, will be spoken to kindly by the other congregants whenever they attend a function. Everyone will be nice and friendly but rarely will they become personal friends. Other people are friendly because they are kind but this is not the same as a personal friendship. When the individual heals and is able to perform volunteer service to others in the congregation, those with whom he or she works on those tasks will treat them more normally. They may well become good friends now that the pity is gone and it's just two individuals working on a task. Even if they do not choose to perform volunteer work, they will be able to be treated as a regular member of the congregation.

How to Begin to Neutralize Your Secondary Gains

In order to neutralize the secondary gains you may be experiencing as a result of the stuff you now want to release, you will need to be brutally honest with yourself. Ask yourself what you are gaining now, how you are gaining it, and how you would like to meet those needs in a more healthy way. You must acknowledge that your needs are being met now in ways you do not want. You are going to have to decide what you are getting from the stuff-related condition, whether it is something you want and, if so, how to continue to get what you want. You will not be able to get what you want all the time, but you are not getting everything you want now, either. In order to get what you are getting, you are not "getting" to be well. You may be getting others to do your bidding or put your needs above their own FOR NOW but this will not last. The other people in your life cannot continue to sublimate their needs and wishes to yours if they are to remain healthy.

If you are using your stuff-induced condition to control conversation, you are going to have to learn or re-learn to engage in normal social interaction again. You will have to learn to give the short, socially appropriate answer, "Fine, thanks" when asked how you are. The more you say it, the more true it will feel. If you realize that you are monopolizing the conversation and you want to stop this inappropriate behavior, your friends and relatives can be enlisted to assist you. Friends and family members can be asked to introduce other topics of mutual interest, such as holiday plans or a bit of juicy local or family gossip, so that you have to share the conversational limelight. This is more normal, more interesting for the other people involved and helps to loosen the hold of the secondary gain.

Maybe your family and friends are doing what you want them to do, even rearranging their own lives in order to cater to your whims. It is fun to be in command, to have others dance to our tune. However, it is not healthy to be achieving this by holding onto stuff that can make you ill. It is also not healthy, let's be honest, to be permitted to run roughshod over other people. Most people will not want to be around someone who does this, though they may feel like insensitive heels if they were to cut off a "sick" person. They will probably just drift away, as this is more comfortable and easy for them if they do not want to continue to dance to your tune. If you are doing this, your need for prominence in your family or group of friends is being met in a nonpermanent, unhealthy way. If you want to begin to unstuff yourself, you are going to have to accept that you will have to take turns being in charge in your group. Sometimes it will have to be acceptable for you to take a backseat and let others be in charge. You will meet your need to run things when it is your turn or by offering to plan and make arrangements for the next activity, in short by doing your share of the work like any other member of the group. This is a much healthier and sustainable way to meet this need.

Maybe your secondary gain is not prominence in your social group. Maybe it is financial. Our society provides financial support for people with medical problems either through public programs like Social Security or through individual means such as increased alimony for a disabled ex-spouse. There is also private disability insurance that people purchase for their own protection. These are something of an incentive for some folks to hold onto their stuff, as they may fear losing this safety net of financial support. You need to remember that these forms of support do not provide a great deal of money or a wonderful lifestyle. They provide basic subsistence income, if that.

Many of these programs are set up in a way that gives the subtle, or not so subtle, message that the recipient is completely incapable of self-support in any form. Social Security Disability, for example, allows "trial" work periods after which the individual is considered eligible to receive benefits, though on a temporarily inactive status, for a number of years. This gives the message that the government believes that people like this individual are useless in the sense of not being able to work or earn money, but that we will indulge them in allowing them to try it anyway. Working is "punished" by a loss of support and health insurance, in the form of Medicare. For people recovering from medical problems, this is a scary proposition.

If you have a skill or profession that you can practice, you can easily earn more than the tiny amount you were receiving for being disabled. This is less terrifying when you realize that even people earning minimum wage usually earn more than Social Security disability payments and nobody can tell you how much to earn or how to spend your money. In fact, even if a family is wealthy and provides total financial support for a disabled member, usually that person loses control of how to spend the money, where to live, what to do and so on. Financial freedom is so much a part of the American psyche that removing it really hurts and offends.

It may seem like a daunting task, but earning your own living in a way that really suits you is a wonderful secondary gain for getting rid of your stuff. Freedom to earn and spend as you see fit is your right as an adult in this society. It is time to free yourself from the infantilizing Big Brother aspect of governmental or other "disabled" financial tyranny! Remember that you can take some time, as you begin to loosen and remove the stuff that made you sick, to figure out what you want to do for work and to train for it.

Many individuals have used the time during which they received financial assistance to train for a new type of work, perhaps one that is easier on the body or more interesting. I used the time I received Social Security Disability payments to train as a hypnotherapist. After I began to practice my profession, I requested that they stop the payments, even though it took considerable argument on my part to convince them to do so. Once you are free of the stuff that caused the medical issues, you still have the new skills and are free to pursue the new profession. These skills may be considered a primary gain, as they do not go away when you become well, and gaining them was made possible as a result of the stuff-generated condition.

Often there are programs that assist recovering people (whom they continue to call "disabled") in finding and paying for training for new professions. Use these programs; you will more than pay for them in taxes as you earn what you like. You know that making use of these types of programs is not the same as staying sick because they were set up to assist those individuals who have used financial benefits to get off benefits. Just because the folks running these programs do not really believe that this is possible does not make it impossible for you!

Relationships with medical personnel or therapists can be a secondary gain as well, difficult though that is for many people to understand. For some individuals whose stuff has made them ill, these relationships become incredibly significant, as they may believe that their care providers are the only ones who will listen to or understand their needs. The friendly and caring attitude of the care providers, which is very appropriate as they strive to help their clientele, may offer the most kind and supportive experience of the individual's day. This is especially true in cases where most personal relationships have drifted away for one reason or another, which happens quite often when a stuff-caused condition creates significant disability. The removal of these relationships is very frightening or feels like a huge loss to the individual who wants to remove stuff and be well.

If you are in this situation, you need to be very clear that although this does feel like a loss of friends, it is not. Paid care providers should never be confused with friends, friendly though they may be. You need to determine ways in which you can replace these relationships with equally satisfying ones. If you enjoy the teacher/student aspect of your relationship with your physical therapist, for example, then maybe a basic exercise or yoga class would be fulfilling for you. It would offer a similar type of teacher/student relationship in a way that is not dependent upon your being unwell in any way. Many, many well people choose to improve their physical fitness by taking such classes, after all. You can be one of them! Who knows, you might actually get fit, lean and gorgeous in the process.

It may help you to consider that each time you are able to stop seeing a care provider, it is like graduating. Give yourself a treat; use the money you used to spend on the provider on something really nice for yourself. If you are able to stop seeing a specialist, use the money you used to spend on travel to the specialist or whatever it cost you for parking and the specialist's time and so on for a manicure or something else you would enjoy. Who knows, you may develop a friendly relationship with your manicurist! Again, this is something you can do as a well person.

For individuals whose stuff has generated recognizable disease there are often disease-related organizations. These organizations offer support and information as well as social activities. Their stated intentions are generally to assist those afflicted with whatever condition they cover. However, they usually keep those individuals in a dependent position. They are virtually never started or run by the affected people themselves, but by "experts" who are generally unaffected themselves.

The social events offered by disease-related organizations are often the only social interaction that some individuals may have. It is vital, therefore, that individuals who want to release their stuff must find alternative and better social interaction opportunities. If other friends and social groups have fallen away while a person is dealing with stuff-related medical conditions, he or she will need to make a real effort to find alternatives. Church and civic organizations are possible choices for ready-made social interactions. Another possibility is to call old friends on the phone and let them know that you are now working on releasing your stuff and could use their assistance in getting back into life. Most likely, they are missing you as well and will welcome you back into their lives, willing to assist you in any way they can. Getting involved in new social activities that interest you is a wonderful secondary gain to getting rid of your stuff. You could actually have some fun!

While participating in disease-related organizations, sometimes individuals make a true friendship connection with other participants. A shared set of experiences can lead to humor and a warm connection between individuals. There is no reason to abandon these friends, as long as they are not holding you back from releasing your stuff. It can even be a shared journey to an extent, just be clear that each individual is on his or her own path and is working on his or her own stuff. If, however, your friend is unhelpful and unsupportive of your choice to get well then it may be time to lovingly release that relationship. If friends are not supportive then they are probably not ready to let go of their own stuff and may feel threatened by the idea that it is even possible. They might be so "married" to the condition that your choice to change that situation in your life is a very scary idea for them. When people are "married" to a condition, that means that it is so much a part of who they are or they are getting so much from it that they are uncomfortable or even fearful of anything that threatens that situation. Their fear reaction can possibly be expressed as anger, maybe they will say that you are being foolish or stupid because they feel that it is impossible for you to get well. Do not get angry with them, they are only afraid. Just let them know that you love them but that you need to take care of yourself right now.

Finding Joy

What is it that gives you joy? I don't mean just what makes you smile or even what you think ought to please you or what is considered good for you, but what gives you huge, enormous, ecstatic JOY! Whatever it is that gives you joy makes you smile, belly laugh, and giggle with sheer delight. It makes you feel like a kid who has been given the keys to the candy store, absolutely transported with happiness and fun. It can also provide you with a sense of inner peace and contentment that fills you right up and leaves no room for unpleasant feelings or thoughts. Only you know what it is, or maybe you do not know that you know yet.

Never mind, you will find your joy and you will know it when you find it. Everyone has something that provides him or her with deep-down joy, and so do you. It is a part of being human. There are a number of methods by which we can find our true joy. You are going to have a great time finding yours!

Many people do not know what their true joy is. They may believe they have nothing that transports them with delight; maybe they think they are too smart or too grown up, whatever that is. They may be feeling too sad or depressed to believe that anything will ever make them laugh out loud again. These individuals are the most in need of finding their joy, though they may not feel able to find it. Friends and loved ones can help by talking about fun times the person had when they were younger or discussing their own joyful activities.

One way to find your joy is to sit quietly for a moment, take a nice, deep breath, and think back to the most fun you ever had. Even if you do not believe you can ever do whatever it was again, just imagine the feeling. Now begin to imagine the things that you think might be your joy...remembering that you can have more than one activity or experience or "thing" as your joy. Apply the feeling from your biggest joy to those other ideas one by one, asking if the feeling fits. If it does, if it is truly a perfect fit, you have found your joy or at least part of it. If not, it is just something that is fun but not your real joy. Keep it, though, since it is a good thing to have fun in your life.

Sometimes the best way is to do a sampling. The way you do a sampling is to try out a whole lot of activities and experiences, some familiar and some brand new, until you find a few that give you pure joy. Ask your friends and family what gives them pure joy, or what is really fun to do. Ask them to share these activities with you, in whatever way you are currently able to do that. Most of the time, people are delighted to share their favorite activities. Enjoy the sampling; it's going to open whole new avenues of fun and pleasure for you. It is OK to have one, two, or many routes to pure joy. The more routes you have, the easier it is to get there when you want.

If you really do not know what would give you unbridled joy and a sampling has not fulfilled your needs or was not possible, it is time for a little research. Go to the library. Look through books and magazines that depict things people do, hobbies, sports, or whatever. Even if you are completely physically unable to actually do the things depicted, look at the pictures or read the descriptions. If you prefer, you can watch TV programs about crafts, painting, and recreational activities of all types. Watch the way people do things and look at the results if there are any. You can also simply watch people in parks or any other place people go when they want to have fun. Observe different recreational and leisure activities in whatever way makes sense for you at this time. With each activity, ask your body for a "yes" or a "no" response. There is a description of how to do this in the section on **the Road to Wellness** later in this book. If your body says "yes" to something you cannot physically do now, that is fine. You can be a spectator, fan or supporter of the activity for now. You can watch or in some other way support or enjoy most activities in which you cannot physically participate now. Perhaps after you have gotten rid of your stuff you will be able to participate in it more fully. A good example of this is dancing. I love to go dancing, but for many years, I could not actually dance at all. I could not stand or move very well and I had poor balance. I could, however, watch and appreciate other people dancing and enjoy the music. Now I can dance and I do, though with a bit less grace and style than I hope to develop in the coming years. Practice makes perfect, after all, and I am very much out of practice.

Exercise Your Joy

For some people, the experience of joy feels foreign. Maybe they have not felt joyful in some time, or they may believe that there is no cause for joy for whatever reason. They may even be so comfortable with depression or sadness that they feel that it would be inappropriate for them to feel joy. For some folks, it seems that the "seriousness" of their condition has them convinced that they should remain serious or subdued at all times. Maybe they have forgotten how to feel joy. If this is the case for you, it may be difficult for you to find your joy since you do not know what it feels like. These simple exercises will provide you with a framework on which to hang your joyful experiences. Remember that Patch Adams said that dying takes two minutes and all else is living!

Pretend that whatever you are doing right now is delightful, really wonderful fun. If you are sitting in a chair and reading these words, pretend that it is the most comfortable chair that you have ever enjoyed and you really love reading about joy. It makes absolutely no difference whether this is true or not; just pretend that it is. Really get into the pretending; snuggle into the chair, and find wisdom and wit in these words. Surely the wit and wisdom is there, after all! Soon you can pretend that you are not pretending and really enjoy what you are doing. Do this with several of the activities you engage in throughout your day every day for the next week. It will certainly make your regular activities more enjoyable. You will have developed a habit of finding joy in mundane activities and, more importantly, you will have developed a familiarity with the feeling of joy. Now you can begin to look for this feeling in other things.

Join a Child who is having a lot of fun. Do whatever is thrilling the little one with as much enthusiasm as you can muster. Be a kid again, doing exactly what the child is doing. Even if it is physically impossible for you to get down on the floor and play with toys, you can participate in whatever way you can. Children are very willing to adapt their play to the abilities of their playmates. I defy you to keep a straight face or sour disposition for long while you are doing this. Children naturally live in their joy, as long as we adults allow that, and they delight in having a big person play with them in their world. Do this as often as possible; it will be good for you and the child at the same time.

Watch the funniest, silliest movie, video, or TV program you can find. It makes absolutely no difference what you choose, as long as it is ridiculous and very good fun in your opinion. If you have not seen a funny movie lately, ask friends or the clerk at the video store, they will be glad to share their favorites. We have all heard the story of the man who cured himself of a serious illness by watching "Three Stooges" videos for days on end. You don't have to go that far, unless of course you feel like it! Just enjoying a silly movie or program, alone or with another person, is enough to give you the experience of joy.

Play with puppies or kittens if you enjoy animals. Their antics are often hilarious and absolutely delightful to watch. As these cute little balls of fluff climb all over their siblings and you, strike poses and fall down you will most likely be unable to avoid feelings of happiness, joy, and even love. Who knows, you might even make a lifelong friend!

Give of your time and talents to others. Everyone has something to give, no matter how disabled they feel they are or seem to be. Tutor a child and see him or her learn new skills that can be life-changing, volunteer to assist in any community organization that matters to you, do whatever your talents and abilities would indicate would be of benefit to others on a personal level. Experience the bond that giving freely of yourself, not your money, to another person can create. Do this often enough and you will feel joy on a regular basis and want more of it in this and other ways.

Pamper yourself. Get a manicure, dress up in your finest clothes or try on lots of beautiful things, get a make-up makeover at a department store, do whatever represents glamour to you. Go with a good friend who will really get into it as well and have a great time. You will find yourself laughing aloud with pleasure as you see yourself looking even better than you remember or expect. Whatever you believe is the most luxury you can afford or imagine, do it. Believe that you deserve it, enjoy it thoroughly, and love yourself enough to give yourself whatever delights you.

Comfort foods can also create feelings of joy. Prepare and enjoy the foods from your childhood, the ones you loved and begged your mother to cook for you. Have a whole meal of childhood favorites, whether it makes a balanced meal or not. Do not do it often, of course, but do it occasionally as a full meal. (Now that you are an adult, you can add vegetables if it seems to you that this would make the meal better, or if it feels like the right thing to do.) You can incorporate many of these favorites into your regular diet, as long as you are somewhat sensible. Very often, just enjoying a taste that brings us back to happy times and places can bring incredible joy, so dig in! It doesn't have to be just desserts. Choose those foods you didn't admit to liking as a kid because they weren't cool, like Brussels sprouts or grapefruit. While proper nutrition is vital for people who are getting rid of stuff, it is also acceptable to indulge yourself from time to time in order to experience joy. You will probably find that many of these favorites are actually appropriate for your body. Children are very wise about what they need and often prefer those foods that are the best for them.

Go out with friends or relatives. Go to a favorite restaurant or bar, maybe one you have not been "able" to visit for a long time. Perhaps you would rather go to a ballgame, theater, or concert. Whatever you pick, it should be the sort of outing you most miss and desire. Because of federal accessibility laws, just about any venue in America should be open to you, so feel free to select what you most want to do. Choose as your companions those people you most enjoy, the ones with whom you laugh the most. Do not invite anyone who will look at you sadly and ask pityingly how you are feeling or if it's "too much" for you.

Treat yourself to whatever you have been denying yourself. Only you know what that means. Maybe it means getting out the good china and eating your peanut butter sandwich off your very best. Maybe it means reconnecting with an old friend or a favorite cousin whom you haven't seen since childhood. Maybe it means something else entirely, something you have stopped doing or that you have never done but always wanted to do. Whatever it is, do it and enjoy it.

Joy spreads itself throughout your life. The more joy you experience in your daily activities, the more you will take care of yourself. Tasks required to provide for your economic or physical well being will seem less onerous as they are just the necessary activities that will provide you with the wherewithal to get into your joy. You will probably even find that these tasks can become fun as you begin to find pleasure, if not true joy, in everything about your life.

Joy is contagious. As you experience joy on a regular basis, it will be natural for you to begin to want to spread it around to all of the people you touch in your day-to-day travels and activities. You will want to share your special treats with those you love, perhaps inviting friends and relatives to do things with you. Joy shared is joy doubled. Most likely, you will find people in your circle who enjoy the same things you do, though each person's individual joy quotient will differ with each activity.

You will also find that, as you experience your special joy in regular doses, you will discover more and more things in your world that delight you. Little things will please you much more than they ever did before. You will notice that you spread happiness through being a more joy-filled person so that even casual interactions such as with supermarket checkout clerks are opportunities to spread a little happiness to others.

People are drawn to happy and joyous individuals, so you may find that some of the secondary gains you used to receive out of pity are offered to you because people feel like they are happy when you are around. Special treatment such as being offered better seats at shows or opportunities to do fun things seem to happen more often to happy people than to morose ones. It is much more appropriate to receive treats for being happy and nice than for being considered in some way damaged!

There is a woman who is usually positive and friendly to everyone she meets, truly finding joy in the smallest things. She calls herself the "queen of the upgrades" because people, from flight attendants to ushers to hotel clerks are always offering her upgrades because they like her. She is so joyous and shares her joy so generously that they want to see her smile even more. It must be said that she enjoys her upgrades and revels in the fun things that happen for her, thus increasing her own joy and the joy she spreads to others. It is a wonderful spiral that continues to provide her with nice experiences.

Like every other skill, the ability to find joy in everything you experience grows stronger the more you use it. The more you allow joy into your life, the more and deeper your joy in whatever happens in the course of everyday living. The more you experience your joy, the more you want to have of it. Therefore, you will find more joy more easily more often. Isn't that a great way to live?

Why Joy?

In American culture, we understand the need for material possessions, fulfilling work, education, housing, and many other things. We do not devote much, if any, time to the search for joy. We have a Constitutionally guaranteed right to pursue Happiness, but we do not even understand why we should undertake such a search. We consider joy, delight, and bliss to be the province of children and the irresponsible. We forget that happy people live longer and are healthier.

Joy causes endorphins—hormones that are much stronger than any narcotic but without the side effects of drugs—to flow in the body. This minimizes or removes pain, anxiety, and stress from the system. Blood pressure stabilizes, metabolism is said to improve, the whole body functions more correctly. Our health literally improves in measurable ways as we become happier.

Scientific studies have shown that even petting a cat or dog, in people who like animals, offers significant health benefits. This activity is simple and often provides a true sense of contentment and inner peace. There is no room for any unpleasant thoughts or feelings. This is also joy, a quiet sort of joy to be sure, but joy nonetheless, and the benefits are obvious.

Joy feels good. This is such an obvious truth that it is often overlooked. It just plain feels wonderful to be happy, filled with delight, and bubbling over with excitement and wonder. Deep contentment feels sublime as well. We tend to discount the benefits of these good feelings, but they are fundamentally important to our sense of well-being as humans.

When we have a healthy amount of happiness, contentment, and joy in our lives, we are able to ride out the inevitable crises that are a part of normal human existence. We are in balance and these events, while distressing, do not fill us back up with stuff. We are quickly and easily able to release the stuff that these experiences give us without becoming ill.

So why Joy? Because it keeps us well.

The Road to Wellness

There are many ways to drive along the road to Wellness, and each individual must choose for himself or herself how far to travel and at what speed. The road is broad enough to accommodate individual differences and choices. Each part of this section will deal with one aspect of the road to Wellness.

Happy Trails!

The Simple Steps to Wellness

As has been discussed throughout the earlier parts of this book, there are a number of simple steps that individuals can take to improve their health. These Simple Steps to Wellness are designed to help any traveler to move along the Road to Wellness more quickly and comfortably. Please use your own intuition and knowledge of your own body to determine how to take these Steps.

1. **Eating** regularly the foods that are most appropriate for your body in appropriate amounts is absolutely vital for wellness. This does not necessarily mean losing weight or attempting to attain some generalized goal for weight. It means nourishing your body appropriately while you are getting well. An interesting experience is that often an individual's weight and appetite will stabilize when proper nourishment is provided. Please note that this is not a carte blanche to eat all sorts of comfort food or junk food all the time without regard to the nutritional value of that food because you think it makes you feel better. It is simply the idea that proper nutrition for your individual body is beneficial. You can discover what the proper food for you is by working with a nutritionist or by asking your body. While enjoying occasional

comfort foods is a joyous experience and appropriate from time to time, keeping an eye on good nutrition is beneficial. After all, good nutrition helps us to be healthy and that is also a joyous experience.

2 **Rest** is extremely important to anyone who is working to get rid of harmful stuff. Good sleep habits are easy to establish if you know how. Every day, whether you have a need to do so or not, get up at approximately the same time. Do something useful or interesting during the day. Get dressed in appropriate daytime clothing every day. If it is at all possible for you, spend the daytime in a different area of your home or go out daily. Go to bed at about the same time each night. Before going to bed, have a warm drink and a soothing bath if you wish. Epsom Salt, bath salts, fragrant bubbles, or essential oils such as lavender may be used to help you relax before sleeping if desired. Never use your bed for watching television or eating, but just for sleeping and sex. If you fatigue easily, take a short nap during the day but do not sleep all day if you can help it.

3. **Water** is essential to good health. Unless there is a medical reason such as kidney disease, drink 8-10 large glasses each day. One way to keep track of your water consumption is to get a mini-cooler that you fill daily and keep in the refrigerator or on your table. These are available in many stores and hold 80 ounces, a reasonable day's target consumption. It is fine to add ice and lemon or lime and to use a straw if this makes drinking all that water easier for you. Please note that soda, tea, coffee, and so on are not

water, even if they are made with water. Do your body a favor and drink the real thing. If you do not like the water in your community, you can put a filter on the faucet or buy bottled water. Whatever you do, drink your water!

4. **Exercise** is beneficial for many individuals. As long as it is medically appropriate for your body at this time, choose a form of exercise you can do. Even people who are not medically permitted to exercise physically can often stretch or do breathing exercise. Sometimes, when regular types of exercise is not permitted, there are options such as Feldenkrais® or similar methods which are taught by physical therapists and other knowledgeable professionals. For myself, when the diagnosis of muscular dystrophy meant that exercise was forbidden, I took a Feldenkrais class taught by a physical therapist I was seeing for other work. In general, exercise is a very important of being well. It stimulates endorphins (the "feel-good" hormones), instigates good breathing patterns, increases the metabolism, and develops overall feelings of well-being. In addition, it is really a lot of fun to notice how much more exercise you can do as you begin to get well.

5. **Participate** in your world. Reach out to friends and family. Make a telephone call just to chat about day-to-day things, not how ill you feel…even if you feel pretty lousy! Ask them about their lives. You will feel better for not focusing on whatever issues and problems you may be dealing with and the person you call will be relieved to have been able to talk with

you about other things. They will be more likely to call you for more conversation after such a positive experience. The more you do normal everyday things, the more you will want to do more of them. This in itself feels good and loosens the hold your stuff has on you.

6. **Mental exercise** is also important to wellness. Depending on your situation, this can be everything from watching a documentary on a subject that is either interesting or new to you to taking a class at a local community education program or university. There is a whole world of thoughts, ideas, and information that you have yet to explore. Feel free to choose anything you like, and to change your mind as often as you wish. Whatever it is you choose, use your mind every day to prevent mental atrophy and to increase your mental wellness.

7. **Emotional or spiritual activity** is also a vital part of wellness. This may mean going to your preferred house of worship, meditating at home or talking with a trusted friend or counselor. For some people it means spending time in nature or with pets. Whatever it means for you, paying attention to your emotional and spiritual health will pay off in wellness now and later on in life.

Asking Your Body

Your body is very wise. It knows exactly what is going on with you and what you need to do for yourself. In order to bring this information to your conscious mind, all you need to do is ask your body.

Everyone's body has a "yes" and a "no" response, which you can use to communicate with your body. This exercise is intended to help you learn what your body's responses are. Please read it through first so that you will understand what you are being asked to do.

To discover what your own "yes" and "no" responses are, close your eyes and get very quiet for a moment. Ask your body to show you the "yes" response and then be aware of what is going on in your body. You will probably experience a flutter or light, happy feeling somewhere in your body. That is your "yes" response. If you have difficulty finding it, do not worry. For many people, the "no" response is easier to find. Again, close your eyes and get quiet for a moment. Ask your body for the "no" response and then be aware of what you are feeling within your body. You will probably experience a dull, tight or heavy feeling somewhere. This is your "no" response.

You can practice this until it is easy for you to find these responses. In time, it will be completely comfortable and natural for you to obtain these responses. For some people it is an immediate "a-ha!" that feels perfect right away. Once you are able to find the responses reliably, you can begin to ask your body all sorts of questions. You can ask it what foods are best for you to eat, what sorts of exercise is best and whether a specific therapy is appropriate for you at that time. You can actually ask your body whatever you want, and you will get answers. Just remember that you will need to phrase your questions so that yes/no responses are possible.

Some psychics and others will recommend using pendulums, which is another way of asking your body because the pendulum works with the impetus of the unconscious mind. Pendulums are an easy way for many people to get their body's answers if they have difficulty feeling the responses. A useful thing to do if you feel the need to use a pendulum is to pay extra attention to what your body is feeling while you are using the pendulum. Soon you will find you do not need a pendulum to communicate with your own body. After all, why should you need a device to communicate with yourself?

To use a pendulum, grasp the pendulum loosely but comfortably in your dominant hand. Ask it to show you a "yes" response. Notice that the pendulum begins to move back and forth in a particular direction, such as forward and back. Now stop the pendulum with your other hand, let it hang still again and ask it to show you a "no" response. Notice that it will begin to move in a different direction, such as left to

right. You can stop it again and ask for a "maybe" type of response if you want. Often people get a sort of circular movement for that. None of these movement directions are absolute, your pendulum might move in very different directions to the ones noted here, and that is fine.

Pendulums are good, but there is another way of getting the information if you are having difficulty "hearing" your body's answers. It is called Kinesiology.

Simply take your non- dominant hand and place the tips of the smallest finger (pinky) and thumb together to make a circle. Now pinch the thumb and first finger of the dominant hand and place this shape inside the circle. Ask your question as you attempt to open the fingers of the dominant hand. See if the dominant hand can break the circle. If so, the answer is no; if not, it is yes. In other words, a strong circle indicates a positive response to your question.

With practice, Kinesiology becomes almost second nature and is used by many individuals to assist them in making choices when they are having difficulty "hearing" their body's answers. However, by working diligently to "hear" the body's answers, soon there is no need to take the time to use even this simple method.

Remembering that your body is incredibly wise, you can see how important it is to set up a dialog with your body. As long as you phrase your questions in a yes/no manner, your body will be able to provide you with answers. Your body stands ready, willing, and able to assist you. All you need to do is ask!

Modalities and Methodologies

There are probably as many modalities and methodologies for traveling the Road to Wellness as there are kinds of cars on the road from Boston to New York. You and your body are wise enough to sift through these modalities and methodologies and select the ones that best suit you. Please remember that your needs may change as you get rid of more and more of your stuff and become more and more well. Just like with those cars, different sizes and styles fit different needs. A family with six children will naturally require different transportation from a single person who is looking for a sexy image. So, too, different modalities and methodologies will be appropriate for different individuals at different times. Whatever is appropriate for you, removing your stuff and finding the road to Wellness will likely leave you a changed person physically, mentally, emotionally, and even spiritually.

As you begin to move toward Wellness and a lowered stuff quotient, remember to continue to experience your joy on a regular basis. Nature abhors a vacuum, so fill the spaces left by the stuff with Joy! There will be no room for the stuff to return if the space is already full.

Choosing the right road to Wellness is an individual task. There are, however guidelines which can assist you in finding your road. These guidelines fall into two categories, Objective and Subjective Guidelines. As you learn about the different modalities and methodologies, which we are calling the roads to Wellness, consider these guidelines and ask your body for the answers to the questions as you go along.

These guidelines are not new or unique. In fact, many of them first appeared in my previous book, **Beyond Disability,** with regard to choosing treatment for a medical issue. The list is somewhat expanded, but the original guidelines are as valid today as they were when that first volume was written.

Objective Guidelines

These guidelines relate to the objective, observable aspects of the road you are considering. They are the things that most people would notice. Remember there are no right or wrong answers; there are just your answers. Some answers will be obvious and some will require that you go within and ask your own body.

1. **Is this road available?** This means that you must be able to find a practitioner or otherwise gain access to the road to Wellness that you are considering. Financial considerations also come into this decision. If the service costs more than you can afford, are you able to arrange something mutually agreeable with the practitioner? Where is the closest practitioner? You might have to make travel arrangements or see the practitioner when he or she visits your area. You will need to make these decisions for yourself.

2. **Is the road a safe one?** What is involved in the modality that you are considering? For some individuals who have significant difficulties due to their stuff, some modalities are too rigorous for their safety and comfort at this time. They may need to get rid of enough stuff another way in order to be healthy

and strong enough for some of these roads to Wellness.

3. **What information can I gather about this road to Wellness?** Ask questions! Research on the Internet or at a library if that is possible for you. Talk to others who have traveled this road. Contact the potential practitioner and ask any and every question that you can imagine. Gather information from any source, as long as you believe it to be reliable. After you have done all of this, you can then evaluate the information to see if it makes sense to you for you. As you review the information, pay close attention to your body's reactions as well as to any emotions that may come to the surface for you.

4. **What is the reputation of the practitioner or organization with whom I will be dealing?** Is it honorable and above reproach? Would I be embarrassed or proud to tell someone whom I respect that I am dealing with him or her?

5. **What is the expected outcome of this particular road?** This relates to the reason you would choose to follow this road to Wellness. What are other people's experiences with using this service to address the type of situation or stuff you are wishing to remove? Is it appropriate or inappropriate for you to even consider this road to Wellness if you really want to remove your stuff effectively? Please remember to ask your body for the definitive answer.

Subjective Guidelines

These guidelines are about the things you cannot see with your eyes or hear with your ears. Only the individual can answer these questions for himself or herself. These intangible, personal issues really do contribute to the success or failure of a modality or methodology. Remember to ask your body, its wisdom will really help you in this area!

1. **As I consider this road to Wellness, how does my body react?** Is there any tightness anywhere or is your body giving you the "no" response we worked on earlier? Do you feel an irritation that seems to come from the pit of your stomach for no reason? If so, just put it aside and move on to another road. If you are getting the "yes" response, continue with these questions. If you are not getting a "yes" response, please research a different modality because this one is inappropriate for you at this time.

2. **What about the practitioner**? Do I believe him or her to be a person with whom I can communicate and in whom I can trust? How do I feel when I am near him or her or when we talk on the telephone? Do I feel that this individual cares about me as an individual or is there a cookie-cutter aspect to his or her

response to me? Pay close attention to your body's responses and your emotional reactions when you talk with the practitioner or think about him or her.

3. **If this modality or methodology is a part of an organization, what is its reputation in my mind?** Am I comfortable with what they espouse and do? Even if they have a reasonably good reputation with others, if your body reacts with a "no" response when you read about the organization, pay attention!
4. **Do I want to travel on this particular road to Wellness with this particular individual?** Even if you like and trust the individual practitioner, do you feel comfortable with him or her in terms of this particular road? A wonderful person who is a terrific practitioner in one area may not be right for you in another. Again, listen to your body!
5. **Am I comfortable with the proposed or projected process?** Find out what the process will be and ask your body if this is acceptable. If you feel a little bit of apprehension prior to a process that might be a bit strenuous or uncomfortable, that is fine. However, if you get a definite "no" response when you consider the process you need to put the process aside for now. If you get a "yes" response, even though you may have some concerns about the comfort of the process it is reasonable for you to consider following through with it. At this point, it is a judgment call on your part.

If you trust your body, your own intuition and your reactions you will be able to select a road as you travel towards Wellness. You will be able to choose your road with comfort and confidence.

Traveling That Road

A Word to the Wise

Now you are ready to remove the stuff that has held you back, stuck in patterns that no longer serve you. That's great! While you are doing this, you need to know that you do not have to drop any of your current practices that support you at this time. Do not stop taking medications without talking to your health-care practitioner because some medications must be reduced and stopped slowly. You may need to continue to take some medications for a while, because your body has become accustomed to them. Be aware of how you are feeling and communicate this. If you are currently receiving acupuncture or other health services, feel free to continue if you want to. With some modalities, you may need to avoid energy work or other types of incongruent treatment for a time. In that case, do what is required.

Working By Yourself

When some individuals choose to get rid of their stuff, they choose to do this by themselves. There are many stories of people who instinctively or intuitively understood what they and their bodies needed do to in order to remove the stuff that was causing them problems. This is certainly one option you have.

If you believe that you would like to work on yourself, ask your body if this is the correct choice. If you get a "yes" response, then ask your body what you need to do to remove the stuff. If you are working with a "yes/no" system as described previously, you will need to phrase the questions in that binary fashion. You can think of all the things you could possibly do and ask your body about them one by one. There may be only one thing you need to do to remove your stuff, or there may be a number of things. It is likely that some of the things will be physical, such as receiving more massages or exercising. Other things you will need to be doing for yourself will probably be emotional, mental, or spiritual. These could include releasing judgment of others, laughing more, engaging in meditation or other spiritual practices or whatever is appropriate for you.

Whatever you determine is needed for you to remove your stuff, be patient with yourself. Give these new activities time to become established and to remove your stuff. Remember that as the stuff becomes less, you may need to add, change, or drop some of these activities. Your body will tell you when this is the case. Listen to your body at all times and you will know what changes to make. Your body is incredibly wise and really does know all the answers. It willingly shares this information if you will only ask.

Working with a Professional

For a great many people, working on themselves is not appropriate or desired. Many modalities require significant training or skills. Generally speaking, a practitioner of some sort is required. Think of this as the chauffeur-driven road to Wellness. You are still traveling the road, but with the assistance of a guide or chauffeur who knows the shortcuts and side streets. Traveling in style like this can be a lot of fun.

Whichever road to Wellness you choose to travel, YOU are in charge. Even when you have a chauffeur, you are still the boss. The issues that are addressed should be those that matter to you. Your agenda is the important one, not the practitioner's. Sometimes practitioners and others have their own ideas of what the agenda should be, and it may or may not be the agenda of the individual who is dealing with removing their stuff. A true professional understands this.

However, when you hire a professional, you need to allow them to do what you hired them to do. If you trust the individual you hired, then discuss the agenda with them. Any responsible professional will be open and willing to discuss with you any issues that are of concern to you. It does not matter what modality or methodology they employ, a professional person should consider the client's needs and wishes when working with an individual on that individual's issues. Your comfort level, physically, mentally, emotionally, and spiritually, is very important. It is never acceptable for such a professional to refuse to discuss these things.

If you do not trust the person you hired to work with you, then you need to ask yourself why you chose to hire that person. What secondary gains are you receiving for working with someone you do not trust, probably paying him or her a lot of money, and most likely failing because of the lack of trust? What are you proving by holding on to your stuff and the problems it causes you? Exactly whom do you believe you are hurting? If you choose to hold onto your stuff, that is your choice and your right, however, you need to really think about why you are paying for a professional if that is the choice you choose to make.

You will be most likely to get the best results if you get your ego out of the way and avoid trying to control or manipulate the situation. This does not mean that you should ignore your red flags if something makes you really uncomfortable. This means that, within the bounds of what you can accept, the professional must do the work in the best way he or she knows how to do it. Maintain an open mind but pay attention to your body's signals.

Once you have met with the professional you have chosen, whether in person, by phone or e-mail, set up the appointments and understood the process, what is next? The financial arrangements must be clear. Know what you are going to be charged and when payment is expected. Make sure you understand clearly what the fees cover and what, if any, other money may be expected later. Are you responsible for the travel expenses if the professional must come to your location? If you must travel, you will almost certainly be responsible for your own expenses. Most professionals are very reasonable about providing this information when asked. Sometimes a professional cannot determine exactly how many sessions may be needed until the work begins and you both see how well your body responds. It should, however be possible to give you a ballpark figure and a per-session fee schedule. Any refusal or reluctance to discuss and be clear about fees, schedules, or services covered should definitely set off your red flags.

Once you have chosen your modality and the professional with whom you wish to work and you have made the financial arrangements you can begin to work. Some modalities for true stuff removal take considerable time and effort. In these cases, it is vital that you understand everything that will be asked of you so that you can get rid of your stuff most effectively. Understanding the time and other commitments that are required will allow you to make whatever arrangements are necessary in other parts of your life.

As you go through the process, regardless of what process you have chosen, issues may come up that are unexpected. The professional should be ready, willing, and able to discuss these issues and to help you work through them. In all probability, the professional will have encountered these or similar issues and will have some suggestions that have been useful to others in your position. These suggestions may or may not fit you, even though they have been useful to others. Before you reject them out of hand, please ask your body if these suggestions are appropriate for you. Do this with each suggestion until you find those that are best for you, and then attempt to follow them to the best of your ability.

Research Tools

There are a number of tools that individuals can use to help them as they search for appropriate modalities, professionals and other resources. These include people you know, the public library, resource directories, televised information and the internet.

People You Know may have had the need for similar services which you now find yourself needing. They have done their own research and determined what was best for their own bodies. They might have had experiences with some of the same professionals with whom you are considering working now. By all means, ask your friends and relatives for their input. If you trust their opinions, or if you know them to be good researchers, you will get good information for your search. However, remember that they might have had slightly different needs and that their bodies are different from yours, even with similar health concerns. If they had a good experience or really liked the practitioner then they could be quite enthusiastic in their recommendations, which might well mean that you will also enjoy that individual. At the very least, it is a good place to start since it is a local recommendation from someone you trust.

The Public Library is a wonderful source of information. You can peruse books, magazines and journals that you might not even know exist until you get there. They usually have a section full of resource books that cannot be removed from the library but can be used there as much as you would like. These books include a variety of types of encyclopedias, medical and other textbooks of the most prestigious sorts and other rare and expensive volumes. You can often gather useful information at your local public library, and materials can be requested from other libraries in your system so the possibilities are virtually endless.

Resource Directories are published in a number of areas. Some deal exclusively with alternative health services and some are more general. Businesses and practitioners purchase space in these directories, so you are not getting a listing of every service that is available in your community. You are getting a list of those who are willing and able to pay for a listing. Therefore, I would not necessarily rely on these directories as my only source of information and names. However, there are two ways in which I would use my local resource directory. I would use it if I had determined that I needed a specific type of practitioner in a specific area or town. If one were listed then I would ask my body if this practitioner was appropriate for me. Also, if I simply needed a list of the types of services that exist, I would use the headings in the resource directory as a starting point. Of course, I could then ask my body if any of the listed practitioners would be appropriate. Sometimes in looking through such a directory, an individual might get a powerful sign from their body that the listing they are seeing is perfect for their needs. If this happens, I would go with it at least as far as making a phone call.

Televised Information usually comes to an individual when they are not expecting it, in the form of a documentary or other informational programming. It might come to you while you are flipping channels looking for something of interest, or you might see a program advertised that appeals to you for whatever reason. The information is seldom unbiased, and it is arranged for maximum entertainment or surprise for the viewers. However, there will be little nuggets that you can use as a starting point for gathering more information as you are searching. Perhaps a program will start you thinking along lines that had never occurred to you before. Ask your body whether the information you are gaining is appropriate for you, and ask it whether you ought to be pursuing this particular line of enquiry at this time. Only you and your marvelous body will know the answer.

The Internet is an amazing source of information on just about any topic you can imagine. There are websites for anything and everything, from breeding frogs to how to bake an apple pie. This definitely includes every medical issue known to man and every alternative therapy anyone has ever concocted. There is no screening process for information on the internet, nor any rules for who may put information up on the net. It is freedom of speech and thought in the most pure form ever conceived and it is wonderful. However, because anyone can put anything out there, the consumer of information must be a bit careful. You cannot believe everything you read, regardless of how nice the website looks. Websites come and go with the speed of light, so what was there yesterday might well not be there today. Certainly you can and probably should do research on the internet, just be aware of the rubbish as well as the good information that is available. If you are not sure about the quality of your information, verify it with a non-internet source or one that you know is trustworthy. As they say, "When in doubt, check it out!"

Living in the City of Wellness

Welcome to your new life in Wellness! You are now free of the majority of your stuff, certainly the part of it that caused you difficulties in the past. While we all have some stuff as long as we are alive, your stuff level is lower than it was, and probably lower than those of most of the people around you. You have worked on yourself in any number of ways, changed the way you do many things and created new relationships in your life.

With all of your newfound wellness, the question arises: what now? Perhaps you have never been well before, not truly as well as you are right now. Maybe the issues with which you were dealing took up much of your time and psychological energy. One thing is clear; you are going to have to learn how to "do" your new life in a way that you can enjoy. You need to figure out how to live in this new space without recreating the stuff that you have just worked so hard to remove.

While each person is different, some truths are pretty close to universal. In order to live in Wellness for the rest of your life, be sure that the Joy you have discovered is a major part of your daily experience. The more Joy, the less room there will be for stuff. Remember that nature abhors a vacuum! You spent a lot of time discovering what gives you joy, reviving the experience of joy and finding new delights. Do not let this go to waste, use this information every day to enrich your life.

When you were burdened with your old stuff, you were not able to do some things and you may have gotten into a routine that was comfortable for you. Another name for a comfortable routine is a rut. Now you can begin to stretch yourself and explore a different way of being and doing. Try new activities and revisit some things that you had given up before you got well. You really must do this because remaining in the boring old rut can trigger body memory and old habits of a less well state. The more you live in a state of health and wellness, the more readily your body and mind will adapt to that new state. The more your body is accustomed to the new state, the more that state will be its baseline or "normal" state.

Other People

The people in your life may have been used to the way you used to be, and now that you are well, they may perceive that you are a different person. They will almost definitely notice that you have changed. They might never have seen you in other than a stuff-filled, ill state. For some people, change is comfortable while others are quite uncomfortable with it.

Your friends and relatives may well feel that their relationship with you has also changed. They are right, at least with regard to some aspects of that relationship. Now that you are able to do things for yourself in ways that may have been difficult in the past, you may well be making choices of which they may not approve. You are living in your joy, doing things that give you deep joy, which you might not have done in the past. Some of your choices might seem a bit unusual to your friends and relatives, and they are going to have to relax and allow themselves to feel comfortable with this. However, the feelings between individuals do not need to change. No matter how your stuff affected your body, your loved ones cared about you, so it stands to reason that your being well need not change that.

While some of your dear ones will be delighted because you are well, others will be likely to feel betrayed or uncomfortable because at least on some level they liked things the way they were. Maybe your stuff-related condition provided them with some secondary gains of their own. For some folks, taking care of a "sick" family member or friend offers the feeling of being needed. Some people subconsciously like the feeling of being in control of some aspect of another person's life, such as what that person eats or driving him or her (and therefore deciding) where that individual might need to go. They clearly had good intentions in that they were willing to assist when that assistance was needed. However, once that assistance is no longer necessary it becomes intrusive. The "helper" no longer has that role and naturally feels some sense of displacement and even confusion. Remember that it is you who have changed, not him or her, so be patient while he or she makes the adjustment to your new persona. For change he or she must, since you are making changes that you have chosen to make and that are in your best interest.

Dealing with the feelings and needs of those who are close to us, especially if they are uncomfortable feelings or needs they do not wish to express, can be fraught with emotional distress. However, it is important to remember that your journey is your own and you are the one who is to make the choices. If others are upset, that is not your issue—it is theirs. Do not make it your issue, though you can help them to adjust to the new reality in kind, gentle, and loving ways.

It is certainly not worth sabotaging your recovery just to keep things on an even keel with the other people in your life. Often people who are recovering from medical conditions, especially those conditions that are stuff-created and considered incurable, will revert to old patterns and recreate their illness because the people who are most important in their life cannot handle the new paradigm. It is sad that these individuals, who bravely faced down their stuff, crumple and fail to maintain their progress in the face of disapproval from (often controlling) friends and family members. You can avoid this problem by being very clear as to who owns your life and what is important to you.

All of the people who have been in your life up until now can have a role in your new life if they are willing to accept your new status. They can help you to find new and wonderful activities that you can now enjoy, as well just being a friend with whom you can share your newfound joy. What they can not do is attempt to control you in any way, especially in ways that would tend to recreate the dependent relationship, if one was present, or put limits on your activities or recovery. You are in charge of your new life, nobody else.

How do we deal with the people in our lives, those who have stood by us and taken care of us when we needed their help? First, we need to understand that it is fear we are encountering. It could be fear of seeing our disappointment when we inevitably (in their opinion) become ill again, fear of loss of role or even just fear of change. Whatever it is, they are truly afraid and we can help them to overcome that fear by being fully in our Joy and bringing them along for the ride. Over time, as we remain well and even get stronger and healthier, the fear of disappointment will probably abate naturally. If these loved ones have a role in our new lifestyle, they should no longer feel any fear of loss of role. If they fear change, then we just need to remind them that we are still ourselves and we still love them. We can engage in old enjoyments, as long as we do not fall into old patterns. For instance, if you and a friend used to watch a certain television program together every week when you were dealing with your stuff-generated issues, you can continue to watch TV together now. This small continuity will probably help them to accept the changes in other areas.

There are a number of strategies which can be useful in dealing with loved ones who are uncomfortable, lost or simply do not know how to cope with the changes you have wrought in your life. You will choose the one that is most appropriate for you in each relationship in which this issue arises. If you are unsure, ask your body.

With some of the people in your life, it is best to confront the issue head-on. Sit them down and tell them what is going on with you. Tell them how the stuff caused your issues and problems. Explain the process by which you got rid of the stuff, and that you believe it is gone permanently. Share with them what you need to do to remain well, and how you are going to take back any aspects of your life that they had been controlling. Do express your gratitude for everything they have done for you and ask that they assist you now in remaining well. They can do this by being affirming in their attitude toward your changes and by enjoying new activities with you as your friend.

There are probably people in your life who will not treat your new wellness and the way in which you achieved it with respect. You know who these individuals are. If they ask what happened, which they might do if the physical changes are dramatic, you can decide how much to tell them. You need to protect your wellness and your confidence in it, yet you may feel strongly about speaking your truth. You can do both by choosing how much to say and in what way. Sometimes an enigmatic smile and a statement that you are fine now is all you will choose. At other times, you might just say that you received some new treatment and are doing well.

There are instances where you will prefer to trust the relationship you have with a skeptical person, and trust that he or she loves you enough to believe you and be happy for you. With those loved ones, take a deep breath, smile, and tell your story. In all probability, you will be pleasantly surprised.

The most enjoyable experiences with regard to dealing with the people in your life will probably relate to children. The children who love you will be so very glad that you are well. If you had been physically ill or disabled, the children in your life will have noticed and had many concerns about you. Children do not understand things in the same way as adults, and are frequently fearful of losing a person whom they love or on whom they depend. They have no skepticism, so when they are told that a person they love is now well they are ecstatic. Their happiness in seeing someone they love "all well again" is a joy to behold!

Another group who will be gratifying when you share your news is the friends who share your comfort with alternative health care. You might want to tell these folks about your healing first, as a sort of dry run with results. These special people will be happy that you are well and glad that something they approve of was involved. They will probably feel vindicated, and therefore be very supportive to you.

Those who love you unconditionally will also be delighted for you because they love you without judging your choices. Even if they feel that the way in which you removed your stuff makes no sense, they will be glad about the results. Unconditional love means that you are loved with no conditions, no limitations, and no expectations of any behavior on your part. I have a dear friend who is very skeptical about anything alternative, yet I know she loves me unconditionally. When I told her about my own removal of stuff and getting well, her reaction was wonderful. She said that if I had chosen to paint myself blue in order to get well, she would have helped me to paint the spots I could not reach. What she meant was that she would support my choices and delight in my new home in Wellness, regardless of how I got there. That is an example of unconditionality that is rare and beautiful.

You, Yourself

You are the most important person in your life. While you are probably concerned with the thoughts and feelings of others, these are of infinitesimal importance when compared with your own. Many of us are taught from earliest childhood that we should try to please others more than ourselves. We do our best to be "people pleasers" regardless of what is our truth. Even if it feels wrong, you must break this habit. This does not mean that you should be rude or nasty, just that you must be true to yourself above all else.

As you remove your stuff, you will begin to feel and function better. Because of this, you will be doing more and different things naturally. You have decided to practice and experience Joy in as many ways as possible as often as possible. These things are certain to change your life in a variety of ways. You have to decide that this is what you want your life to include. It is your life, and therefore the choices that you make for that life are up to you and nobody else.

Be very careful to make changes that you are happy to make and with which you can live. If you are not happy with the changes in your life, you can rest assured that your body and unconscious mind will recreate your stuff. This will recreate your previous stuff-caused conditions, or similar conditions. You will be right back where you started. If this starts to happen, look at the changes you have made and review them one by one. Ask your body whether each change is appropriate for you at this time. Your wise and wonderful body holds the answers, just ask the questions.

Clearly, you prefer to be free of your stuff and the conditions it caused. You have done a lot of work and learning to rid yourself of it. You did all this work because you wanted to remove the stuff and change your life. In order to avoid recreating it, be absolutely certain that the new things you are doing, the changes in your life, are those you want. Make sure that you are doing what you want, not what you think others want you to do. If you are going to get well just to go back to an unhappy existence in some way, your body will recreate the previously successful escape route.

You may remember our lady who developed a stuff-related disability and could no longer do all of the laundry and housework for her family on top of her job. Her family did their fair share of the work and she was able to take care of herself and get well. If, however, she were to get well and have to shoulder that huge burden again, it would no longer be beneficial for her to be well. Her body and mind would recreate her stuff and her illness, as that had worked very well to get her out from under that burden in the past. The body is very smart and learns from past experiences, after all. After she got rid of her stuff, she sat down with her family and discussed an equitable distribution of labor in their home. She retained her ability to take care of herself and do some of the things she wanted to do, and her family members learned to look after their own needs. Everyone benefited, the mother by not recreating her disability and the rest of the family by developing some improved self-care skills.

You are now living in the wonderful city of Wellness. The possibilities are limitless for you to learn and do new and delightful things. Perhaps you can now do things that were physically impossible for you only a short time ago. Maybe you can concentrate better now that you are not taking certain medications, so learning new skills is easier. What do you want to do? Only you can know. Ask your body whether each new opportunity would be beneficial to you. Your wonderfully wise and healthy body knows the answers.

You can possibly learn new job skills that will provide you with a higher level of earning and a more pleasant lifestyle. If this is something that you want to do, you are now in a better position to change your career, as you are healthier than you have been in a long time, possibly your entire life. You have just completed a remarkable task, that of removing your stuff. In doing so, you gained new confidence and skills that will stand you in good stead when you begin to learn the new job skills that now interest you.

Maybe you are satisfied with your professional life. What else can you now do with your new wellness? You are now able to make whatever choices are appropriate for you. If you are fortunate in your professional life, then your choices will probably relate to your personal, social, and recreational life. Because you are now well, there will be a certain amount of adjustment in your perspective. You have adapted to your stuff-created condition and planned to accommodate it in anything you chose to do. Now you can stop doing that and it feels strange, wonderful but strange.

Perhaps you enjoy museums, and have visited many of them, maybe in a wheelchair recently. Maybe you have not been able to go at all due to your stuff and the conditions it has created. Now you can attend galleries and museums if you wish, possibly for the first time in years. If you visited the museums in your area in a wheelchair, you now need to get used to doing so on foot. You will be able to get closer to the exhibits, certainly, as they are arranged for people of the usual height who are standing. You will not be offered special assistance or other accommodations, but now you do not need that sort of help. You can go at whatever time of day suits you or your companions, rather than accommodating limited energy stores or medication schedules.

Making New Choices

So many new choices present themselves now that you are living in the City of Wellness. These activities are intended to assist individuals in understanding how to make these choices.

1. **Professional Choices** are very important. Now that you are significantly free of your stuff and any condition that it may have caused, you are more able to engage in interesting professional activities. You are going to need to support yourself, perhaps, and now you can choose from a plethora of ways of achieving that goal. You have certain levels of training and education, as well as specific talents and interests. These attributes will form a base of information from which you will make your choices. In order to begin to make some of the professional choices, you can do the following tasks:

   a. Make a list of all of the jobs or professional activities that you know exist. Do not limit the list to specific jobs, but include activities that are parts of jobs such as "speaking in public" or similar activities. Think about the professional activities that you have done as well as those that you are aware that other people do. Make the list as extensive as you can. Don't be concerned about whether a specific entry is a "whole real" job or not or whether you are trained for that specific job. Many professional activities include aspects of others, so you are probably qualified for a profession that includes some aspects of many of the professional activities on your list. In addition, training is available for many professions and activities that you might like. Go down the list asking your body which ones are appropriate for you. After you have crossed out the professional activities that are inappropriate for you, look carefully at the remaining options. Feel free to choose any of these which looks like something you would like to do and explore it fully. Determine if you are already skilled in this area, or what training you would need. Determine the employment potential of this area and perhaps begin to make enquiries.

b. If you already have a profession that you enjoy, but that you may have been away from, now is probably the time to return to it. If you have been away from your profession for many years as a result of your stuff-generated condition, your knowledge may need to be brought up to date. In most professions, there are changes that occur over time. These changes might relate to technology, modern ways of interacting with clients, rules and laws or many other things. You will need to find out what changes have taken place and become current with the new information. A nice way to begin is to take a former colleague out to lunch.

You might also be able to check professional journals or organizations, whatever is appropriate in your profession. If you have been receiving disability income of any sort or have been classified as disabled, many states will offer assistance with rejoining the workforce. Go ahead and use this assistance, your tax dollars will soon more than repay the value of what you receive.

c. If you have worked throughout the time that you were dealing with your stuff, that is wonderful! You might feel that you are now ready to take on new challenges either in your current work situation or in a new place of work. If you have been the "disabled worker" at your current place of employment, you will need to assess for yourself whether management and coworkers are able to view you in a different light now that you are well.

2. **Personal Choices** are now available to you that you may have thought were impossible just a few weeks or months ago. You can probably do a wide variety of activities that are new and exciting to you. Your relationships might have changed now that you are well. In so many areas of your personal life, new choices present themselves daily. Doing some of these tasks will probably help you to figure out what you want to do in your own personal life.

   a. Just as you did with professional activities, make a list of all of the activities that you know people have to do to manage their personal lives. This will include self-care activities, cooking, shopping, paperwork, and so many more activities. Perhaps you are not yet able to take over all of these activities, and perhaps you live with others who can and ought to do their fair share. Go down the list, asking your body whether each one is appropriate for you at this time. After you have crossed out the ones that are inappropriate, look at the list and decide if you feel you ought to be responsible for all of these tasks or if others in your home ought to be doing some of them. It is probably time for you to shoulder an appropriate amount of the workload, so please choose your tasks from the list of those activities that your body tells you would be acceptable for you at this time.

b. Romantic relationships are a very important part of anybody's personal life. Very often, when individuals are dealing with the unpleasant results of stuff they avoid these types of relationships. Many people feel that they are not well enough or attractive enough for dating. It is unlikely that your stuff made you unattractive, though you may not have felt well enough to go out on dates. At the time that you were coping with the results of your stuff, you might well have felt that dating would use up too much of your energy. However, now that you are living in the city of Wellness, your energy has probably increased to the point that you can date if you choose to do so. If you are already in a relationship, a marriage for instance, you will most likely find that your new state of Wellness will allow you to revitalize the romantic side of that relationship. What a wonderful secondary gain from removing your stuff!

c. Leisure time activities are another area that improves the quality of life for most people. It is likely that some of the things that you used to like to do before your stuff got in the way were impossible or difficult for you while you were dealing with the results of that stuff. Now you can choose whether to engage in those activities again. You do not have to do anything you don't want to do. If, for example, you enjoyed roller-skating when you were well in your teens but now you are older and it just does not appeal to you, don't do it. While roller-skating is an obvious example, there may be a number of activities that you are not sure about doing after many years. In these cases, ask your body.

Nancie's Story

I was born on February 21, 1959 in Leominster, MA, the first of four children. Although nobody knew it at the time of my birth, I was born with a rare form of muscular dystrophy called mitochondrial myopathy. This condition would later prove to be very disabling, requiring the use of a scooter-style wheelchair and other adaptive devices. I experienced a significant degree of pain and weakness for the first forty-four years of my life. It was primarily a result of critical mass stuff, beginning before my birth and continuing until I unstuffed myself.

My parents were young, college-educated people of Eastern European Jewish heritage. My father was an English teacher at the local high school and my mother was trained as a chemist, though I have always thought of her as a singer. I was their first child, born nearly four years after their marriage.

Both of my parents are atheists, and they raised their four children as such. I cannot speak for my siblings, but I continue to consider myself an atheist. This means that I do not believe in any deity, but it does not mean that I do not believe in spiritual values such as love, joy, and compassion. I do. This is important in understanding my story.

I believe I was an unusual child in many respects. I was a very verbal and observant child, or so my parents have told me. I did not have any idea how other children act, what they say, and so on; so I merely developed at my own pace. As an only child for the first four years of my life, I spent a lot of time with adults. Most adults spoke to me as if I was an intelligent human being, not a baby, and I responded to this as any intelligent child would. I was not a particularly physical child; I didn't climb on the furniture or break things. I preferred to play with toys, talk to adults and so on. I remember a very rich imaginative life as a young child.

Some aspects of my personality were decidedly unusual. For one thing, I have a very full memory of most of my life, from infancy. For a long time I thought that everyone could recall his or her whole life with clarity, and was quite surprised to find that this is not common. In addition, I have always been able to ask my body questions when making decisions, and I receive answers that lead to correct choices. At the age of two, I was able to ask my body about the sorts of simple choices that children make. I came to rely on my own body more that on what others told me, though I used that information as a sort of database.

I was very fortunate to be born into a family that was large, loving and accepting of individual differences. I received unconditional love from my parents, grandmothers, and great-grandmother. I did not know a grandfather, though one lived until I was 27 years old, and I never really missed that relationship. I had a number of great-aunts and uncles as well. There are, of course, family members who were not and are not good and loving but my parents never felt any need to expose their children to these individuals. As a result, my memories of family are colored with love and acceptance.

One of my earliest significant memories took place when I was approximately one year of age. I vividly remember the event. I was in my crib and heard a voice that sounded like an adult tell me to jump up and down in the crib, which I had never done before. The "Grownup," as I dubbed the voice, told me I could get away with jumping because my grandmother was coming to visit and my parents would believe that I was excited. I did not understand why this would excite me as I saw her frequently. Still, it sounded like fun and I did as I was told.

I took hold of the top of the barred area and began to jump. I jumped until my legs shook and I fell down. The Grownup then told me that this was called "fatigue" and that I would have it happen to me for a long time. I remember thinking that this did not sound like a great idea, but that I had no choice.

After this experience my Grownup spoke to me occasionally, generally when I wanted to understand some aspect of human behavior. I must admit that I found the adults around me to be a bit silly and incomprehensible, but I suspect that this is not unusual. Many children seem to have some memory or understanding that does not fit perfectly with what we think of as normal human life. In addition, children are not adults and tend to understand things differently because of having less experience and understanding of the adult world.

As I was developing as a young child, I sometimes had to make choices as to what I would do. These situations are common for children, things like eating a specific food or touching a certain object that could be unsafe. I learned very young, probably before age two, that my body would tell me what would be in my best interest. I got an uncomfortable feeling in my lower abdomen if "no" would be the proper choice and my "yes" response was a fluttery feeling in my upper abdomen. If I ignored a "no" response, the tight, uncomfortable feeling would intensify and even develop into a headache as well until I did respect it. I relied upon these responses throughout my youth and, in fact, I still do.

From the time I was about eighteen months old until I was five, we lived in Fitchburg, MA, in a three-family apartment building. At the side of the house was a wall facing the parking area and play area. I remember one particular day when I was three. I was sitting on the wall when a dog walked across the play area. The dog did not come near me or bother me in any way. It glanced at me briefly. I looked at the dog, I saw something out of the corner of my eye. Looking to the right, I saw a word written in red and purple writing above my right shoulder. This word was one that I, as a child of atheists, had never heard and did not know before that day. This word was "Satanic" and I was able to read it without difficulty. I somehow understood what the word meant, though I had never been exposed to the idea of Satan, Heaven and Hell or any other concepts common in Judeo-Christian religions. I was only three, but from that moment on, I was able to read whatever I saw. I understood the word, understood that it pertained to the dog and ran into the house. I refused to come out for six months and only left the house under duress. To this day, I cannot tolerate dogs at all, and the feeling is definitely mutual. Even very "nice" dogs (which I think is an oxymoron because I have never met one) seem to hate me.

From that moment, I could read as well as any adult. My father was a teacher, and educational theory of the time was that children should not learn to read until the first grade. When I demonstrated that I could read, my parents said it was not real reading, that I could not read until first grade and that I had probably memorized the story. I was a fairly timid, compliant child, so I did not allow anyone to catch me reading.

On the first day of first grade, I probably drove my poor parents crazy asking if I was really starting first grade that day. I asked the teacher, a lovely young first-year teacher, if this was really first grade. She said it was and gave me the primer, the first book I felt I was permitted to read. She probably told me that I would be reading that book; I believe that is what she said. I took the teacher at her word and read the book from cover to cover immediately. It was not exactly a gripping tale, but the sense of freedom at being allowed to read it was absolutely intoxicating. The teacher watched me read it and asked me questions about the characters and the story. She called my mother and chewed her out for teaching me to read-after all my parents had done to prevent it! My mother, to her eternal credit, threw up her hands, went out the next day, and bought me two **Nancy Drew** mystery books. These books are on an upper elementary school level, approximately, and I was able to read them with ease and interest. They were reasonably age appropriate and I thoroughly enjoyed them. A lifelong love of reading was born. I got my first library card the next day and I believe I read every interesting book in the children's section over the course of first and second grade, after which my family moved.

The incident with the dog, which led to my ability to read, was, I believe, a very unusual one. Although I let a fairly normal existence for a little girl of the era, I had other experiences, which, I later learned, were decidedly unique. As I grew older, I became aware that these experiences were not in the normal experience of my friends so I chose not to talk about them. Fitting in, which I could never quite feel that I achieved, was important to me, so I kept my "weird" abilities and experiences to myself.

One experience that I remember clearly happened when I was about three or four years old. I remember sitting on a cedar chest in our apartment in Fitchburg and going into a sort of trance state. In this state, I experienced my life up until the age of eight. My Grownup then told me to go back and live it. I returned to full consciousness, still sitting on the trunk. My life unfolded for the next few years exactly as I had experienced it that day. Every detail was precisely what I had experienced. I remember getting to the end of the time I had experienced and feeling a bit frightened because I did not know what would happen next.

I never told anyone about these experiences. In fact, I went to great pains to hide any differences. Why did I do this? After all, young children do not generally know that their experiences are unacceptable or weird to the broader society. However, I had a very good reason to hide my peculiarity. We had neighbors who were "born again"

Christians. I played with their child. When I told my friend some of my experiences, she told me that it was the work of the devil. I had no clue who or what she was talking about, so she explained that the devil was a very bad creature who would pull me down under the ground into a bad place. As an atheist child, I had no frame of reference for all of this and I did not connect it to the "Satanic" word I had seen. The mental image I remember getting was the Troll from my ***Three Billy Goats Gruff*** picture book pulling me through the hardwood floor. I thought that that would have to hurt and I did not like the idea of it at all. I had the idea that this assault was imminent if I did not stop having "weird" experiences, and that this creature would know whether I did or not. That is enough to stop any little kid from doing almost anything, I would imagine.

Of course, I did not have the ability to stop the unusual experiences of my life; I simply pretended they were not happening. I cannot actually say that this strategy was wildly successful in that nothing changed other than my comfort level with my experiences. Up until this point I was completely unconcerned about these sorts of things, they were normal to me. Afterwards, I was very uncomfortable but felt that it was something I needed to hide and deal with myself.

As I grew up, I continued to get "yes" and "no" responses from my body. I learned to obey these responses because every time I did I benefited in some way. Whenever I ignored the responses, two things happened. The responses continued to grow stronger as long as the situation existed. The other thing that happened was that I did not succeed or benefit from the situation.

Relying upon these responses, I managed to stay out any real trouble as a child and teenager.

I found that I could use my body's responses in my schooling as well. If I was not sure of the answer to a question on a test, for example, I would ask my body and get the response. This was successful because the "yes" and "no" responses are a communication from the unconscious mind and the unconscious mind keeps a record of everything we see, hear, read, experience and learn. It will provide this information upon request, as long as it understands what is wanted. I did well in school, having difficulty only when I did not bother to ask my body or thought I was sure of information that I did not consciously remember correctly. I went through a time where I thought that asking my body was cheating, but I soon realized that all of the other students had bodies they could ask and if they did not do so it was not my fault. Therefore, it was not cheating and I went back to asking my body. It was easier than working hard!

As I said earlier, I was born with mitochondrial myopathy, a rare form of muscular dystrophy. My experience at about age one with my Grownup included an experience of fatigue in my legs, a feeling that became increasingly familiar throughout my life. I had some fatigue and mild discomfort from time to time over the next five years or so, but nothing was so terribly painful that I had to tell my parents about it.

On Thanksgiving Day when I was six years old, my father decided that I was old enough to go to a football game with him. It was a chilly but sunny day and there was quite a lot of walking, standing, and moving involved.

I enjoyed the game, but began to experience significant pain in my legs, which spread to other areas of my body. By the time we left the stadium, I was unable to walk and had to be carried home. At home, I continued to have a lot of pain for the rest of the day. My parents and relatives attempted to behave as if nothing were wrong as they felt it was either behavioral or simple tired legs from doing too much. I remember feeling that nobody noticed the problem and that I should not let others see that I had a problem. Nobody said anything that led me to this conclusion; it was just my six-year-old interpretation of the situation and the responses of the adults around me.

After the age of six, I had frequent experiences of pain and fatigue in various muscles. It had been discovered when I was about four that I have completely flat feet. I wore corrective shoes, which did little or nothing to alleviate the main problem, though they probably helped me to walk more comfortably. I did my very best to do the things my friends did. I took dance lessons, went swimming, walked to the local shopping area, and played ball games. I really preferred sitting quietly and reading, since it caused me no pain. However, I was determined to be a "normal" child, though I knew full well that in many ways this was impossible.

The summer I was thirteen I was a counselor-in-training at the local day camp that I had attended since the age of nine in our new hometown of Mt. Kisco, NY. One of the activities we had was a group camping trip. A part of this trip was a hike in the woods. I was a bit sore but did not listen to my body because I was thirteen and all the cool kids were going on the hike. My body began to hurt so much that I thought I would go insane. In addition, my legs stopped working properly and my whole body seemed to become ineffective. It got so bad that the hike was curtailed and one of the adult guides went back for a vehicle to transport me home where my mother put me in a warm bath in an attempt to relieve the pain. My parents took me to the doctor the next day but no medical treatment was recommended. I eventually recovered, though I had several significant episodes of pain and fatigue throughout my teens.

My parents were not inattentive. They were excellent parents who were unconditional in their love and provided their four children with the most individually appropriate start in life possible. However, when I was a child there were no tests for the type of condition I had and pediatricians did not even do routine blood work on children who appeared reasonably healthy. The physicians my parents chose were well-qualified pediatricians. They suggested that I was experiencing "growing pains" but I firmly believed then and believe now that nobody would grow if it hurt that much. The simple fact of the matter is that I appeared healthy most of the time and medical science had not yet discovered any test or treatment for mitochondrial myopathy. At the time of this writing, there are diagnostic tests but still no treatment.

I was slightly overweight as an adolescent and it was suggested that my pain and fatigue would go away if I lost weight. The summer before I started high school I lost the approximately ten pounds that my doctor considered the cause of my problems. It made very little difference, though it boosted my self-esteem at that tender age.

Because I did not have any sort of diagnosis, I was required to take physical education and participate in the normal experiences of middle school and high school. It was extremely difficult in many ways and may have caused some muscle damage, but it benefited me psychologically to be seen as normal. In middle school, the students were required to jog twenty times around the gymnasium. I lied about how many times I ran. I jogged slowly for a time that was about as long as the average student ran and then I stopped, pretending that I had counted twenty laps. I believe I usually managed between one and six laps. I attempted the twenty laps just once, and it was incredibly painful, so I never did it again.

When I was seventeen, my family went to London because my father received a Fulbright-Mellon teacher exchange. I met and married my husband Timothy during that year, when I was eighteen. I worked in human services in the London Borough of Lambeth from November 1976 through August 1977. That was a pivotal year in many ways, but the "weird" experiences and physical pain and fatigue continued.

Upon our return to the United States, I attended Brandeis University for one year. Deciding I preferred to work, I returned to human services. With my husband, I ran a group home for mentally ill adults who were learning to live outside of institutions. I also worked in the adult education and medical departments of a state institution for people with mental retardation. Although my problems and difficulties continued, I was able to cope with the work although the physical demands were sometimes overwhelming for me. Because of my auditory intuitive abilities, I could understand the often-difficult speech of the individuals with whom I worked. This was very helpful and I allowed my supervisors to exploit my ability as it was to the benefit of the clients. Besides being able to understand their speech better than most other staff members, I used my body's "yes" and "no" responses when I was not sure or needed to make a split-second decision to safeguard the clients' health or comfort.

During my tenure at the institution, I gave birth to both of my children. Johannah was born in 1980 and Samuel in 1982. Physically, my pregnancies were difficult as I experienced increased fatigue due to the extra weight. I was easily able to give birth without medication or any hypnosis training, probably due to my lifelong practice and increased ability to dissociate from the discomfort of my body.

In approximately 1981 my closest friend and co-worker at the institution in which I worked was a wonderful gay man called Jim. Jim was funny, bright, and kind. He treated the elderly, mentally retarded women with whom we worked with respect. Unfortunately, he was diagnosed with AIDS in the mid-eighties. Jim died a painful, horrible death in 1992.

I was fortunate in discovering that a wonderful education in human services could be obtained at the University of Massachusetts' College of Public and Community Service. I therefore stopped working and went back to school. It was a competency-based degree program for adults, and I graduated with a double major in Management of Human Services and Gerontology within three years.

My family and I relocated to Virginia in 1990. I continued to have significant physical pain and difficulty. My "weird" experiences continued as well. I selected our first two homes in Virginia by listening to my body. My husband chose the third, in which we live at this time, and I agreed because the house definitely received a "yes" response from my body.

In 1992, I returned to Boston to visit my dear friend and former co-worker Jim as he lay dying in his apartment. His mother and many friends were caring for him. We had a quiet conversation as Jim could barely speak. I had brought some jelly donut-holes and mocha coffee, Jim's favorite snacks in his healthier days. As I hand-fed Jim, he looked at me. His eyes showed his intelligence and his understanding of his situation. Jim died ten days later.

In Jim's memory, my family worked with the Names Project, commonly known as the "AIDS Quilt" group. We created Jim's Quilt panel together as a family, with the help of a mutual friend. A few months after Jim's death, we were preparing for a large display of the Quilt in Washington, DC. As I worked alongside people with AIDS, I noticed that they could do more physically than I could with less pain or fatigue. I immediately made an appointment with our family doctor.

Significant medical testing ensued, culminating in a muscle biopsy operation. The resulting diagnosis was mitochondrial myopathy, a condition of which I had never heard. I took the diagnostic sheet to the public library, where I looked it up in a medical dictionary, where I saw the words "muscular dystrophy" for the first time. I double-checked in several reference books with the same result. Once I got over the shock, I called the doctor for final verification, which I received.

At last, I knew I was not crazy, and that I needed some assistance. I went to a specialist and got a prescription for a scooter wheelchair and many painkillers with names right out of a science fiction movie. I stopped working eventually, stayed home with my children, and received Social Security Disability payments. I must confess to a situational depression that lasted about three months. Then I got bored and actually filled the prescription for the wheelchair.

After a time, I received a brochure for a weekend seminar on hypnosis. I decided to attend and discovered that this was a field I could enter without needing to walk at all. The father of modern hypnotherapy, Dr. Milton Erickson, was a polio survivor who used a wheelchair at times during his life. If he could do it sitting down, then so could I!

I love hypnotherapy; it is a wonderful profession. Although it was legal for me to work as a hypnotherapist after only fifty hours of training, I enrolled in a great many other, more advanced, training programs and eventually obtained a Doctor of Clinical Hypnotherapy Degree. I joined a number of professional hypnotherapy organizations, in order to continue to learn and improve my skills, as well as having some way of demonstrating that I was a competent therapist. These organizations have educational requirements for joining and annual renewal requires a number of hours of additional training and education each year. At the time of this writing, there is no licensure available for hypnotherapists in any US state, so the organizations do their best to fill that need for hypnotherapists and the public.

Hypnosis organizations usually have annual conventions or conferences. The National Association of Transpersonal Hypnotherapists is no exception. I attended my first NATH convention in Virginia Beach, VA, in 1996. I was sitting in my scooter wheelchair when a blonde woman of about my age approached me. She said her name was Patti and that her husband was in a wheelchair and she was wondering what brand of chair I was using, as they were interested in buying a power scooter. As I shared my information, I had no idea that this seemingly chance meeting would eventually change my life.

I continued to work as a hypnotherapist, having "weird" experiences and weakening physically over the next seven years. I wrote my first book, **Beyond Disability,** and began to lecture at national hypnotherapy conferences. I traveled all over the United States with my wheelchair, both for business and for pleasure. I purchased equipment so that I could visit friends and relatives in England, as well as specialized equipment to allow me to function independently at home.

I also saw Patti at several conferences, always enjoying her company. I attended every class she taught at the conferences. I learned that her full name was Patti Conklin and that she is a medical intuitive. The term *medical intuitive*, in this instance, means that Ms. Conklin is able to see into the human body and move energy in order to assist individuals in healing themselves. For further information, you can see her story later in this book. For several years, we continued to meet at conferences.

It is a sad fact that so many of the individuals who work in alternative health will push their services or products, in the apparent belief that they know what others need. This is especially true when they see someone in a wheelchair or with a visible disability of any sort. I certainly experienced this. I have been poked with crystals, hit over the head with copper objects, and annoyed in countless ways. This sort of inappropriate behavior happened whenever I ventured into the sales rooms at the hypnotherapy conferences I attended or when I went to alternative health fairs of any type. I consistently avoided anyone I thought might treat me with that sort of disrespect. I always refused their offers because it was clear to me that that kind of intrusiveness was something I could easily do without. If the individuals offering services could not respect my "no" then they would not be likely to listen to anything else I had to say. Using the Subjective Guidelines we have discussed, I chose not to use the services of anyone who had difficulty respecting my boundaries.

Patti Conklin never pushed her services on me, but was always respectful of my boundaries. While we met at many conferences and conventions, we generally discussed topics unrelated to my disability. Because of this, and the respect I developed for her as I watched her work during lectures and seminars, I was able to approach her when it was appropriate for me to remove the muscular dystrophy.

In May of 2002, I tested the waters by suggesting that we work together. When Patti began to explain how to make an appointment, and which of her services she felt was appropriate, I began to back off. Clearly, I was not ready. Patti immediately dropped the subject and introduced me to a colleague she had just met. The next time we saw one another, we chatted about a variety of topics and the subject of working together did not come up.

In February of 2003, Patti and I both attended the American Board of Hypnotherapy conference in Newport Beach, California. After Patti gave a lecture, I went over to her and said, "Patti, it's time for us to work together." She looked at me and told me that I was right. She gave me her card and explained how to make an appointment for a *Cellular Cleansing*, which is the service she recommended. I felt no resistance at all. I could hardly wait to get home to make the appointment!

After I returned to Virginia, I began an e-mail correspondence with Patti Conklin. We discussed the cellular cleansing, what it was, what it would be like, and what I could expect from it. I perused Patti's website, listened to her online radio program and learned all I could about her and her work. As the date of the cellular cleansing approached, I became more excited and more convinced that I would benefit greatly from it.

In April of 2003, I flew to Atlanta for my cellular cleansing. The appointment was for 6:30pm-9:00pm on April 8 and 10-4 on April 9. I spent the day of the eighth with a friend who lived in Atlanta. I was ready and waiting when Patti arrived and we began to work.

The Interview

In June of 1004, I was interviewed by Antoinette Attell, a columnist from Los Angeles, CA. Ms. Attell is a performance artist who has received three California Arts Grants to perform mime and comedy for special populations including people with a wide variety of disabilities. The following is an excerpt from that interview.

Can you describe the moment when you first knew that you were ready to be really unstuffed and get well?

Yes, I find it sort of amusing to be honest. It was no great epiphany or anything like that. I simply found that I didn't want to deal with the muscular dystrophy any more. I began to become irritated, not at the usual things like inaccessible stores and rude people but with the actual experience of sitting in the wheelchair. This had never bothered me before as I simply accepted this situation and believed that it was a fact of my life, like having brown hair. However, now I felt like it would be so much more convenient and appropriate to walk and do things for myself. It wasn't a longing for what I no longer had, but it felt like an eagerness to regain what was rightfully mine.

What was the thing that prevented you from healing?

The thing that most prevented me from healing, apart from needing some guidance as to how to do it, was fear. I had not been well for a long time and for a long time I felt some fear over whether I would be able to live that way. I was a bit afraid to attempt to live without my devices and secondary gains. The way I expressed it was that I had never met Healthy Nancie.

How long did you have muscular dystrophy and when was it diagnosed?

Muscular dystrophy is the name given to any one of forty congenital neuromuscular diseases. That means that it is present from birth, though in my case it was not really apparent until later. I had my first experience with muscle fatigue at age one and my first significant pain experience at the age of six. Medical testing for the type of issues I had did not exist when I was a child. When I was 33 years old, I decided to get checked out to find out why I was having such struggles to do the physical things others could do so easily. That was when I had the various tests and the muscle biopsy which led to the diagnosis of mitochondrial myopathy muscular dystrophy. I guess the short answer to your question is that I had it for 44 years and it was definitively diagnosed when I was thirty-three.

Did your mind and body immediately believe the medical diagnosis and fall into the pattern of having muscular dystrophy? When you were diagnosed did your condition worsen and did you fall into that belief system?

Yes, I actually went into a brief period of depression when I learned the diagnosis. I believed that the medical diagnosis was tantamount to a certain fate that I did not want. I worried about my children, about how they would manage with a "sick and useless" mother as they grew older. I stayed in that state for about three months, but then I got bored and filled the prescription for the wheelchair and got on with life.

After that point, I can't honestly say that my condition worsened more rapidly. In fact, it might have improved or at least worsened more slowly because I began to rest more and I took better care of myself. I certainly believed that I had this terrible disease which would eventually rob me of my choices, my abilities and finally my independence.

What would you say was the greatest challenge as a mother with a disability?

That's a tough question, Antoinette. Fortunately, I did not receive my diagnosis until both children were past the stage of needing to be carried and cared for in a physical sense. As a mother I wanted my children to be able to rely on me when they needed help in any area of life. I also wanted them to feel free to leave home to go where they might need to go in order to gain education and follow their dreams. I worried that my medical condition might make them feel afraid to leave or afraid to "trouble" me with their needs as older teens or adults.

What would you say was the greatest challenge as a wife with a disability?

I have a wonderful spouse. Many people told me to be extra nice to him after my diagnosis because the sad fact is that more men leave wives who become disabled than stay with their wives. Women tend to stay but men do not. I didn't listen and didn't change the way I related to my husband at all. I think the greatest challenge is keeping the relationship on an equal footing and making sure that both partners are comfortable with the changes as they occur. This takes some work and a lot of open communication.

What would you say was the greatest challenge as a professional with a disability?

One of my biggest challenges involved making ADA required changes in minor tasks in a County job. Later, working for myself, I had no difficulty with my clients, my colleagues or other professionals. My Chamber of Commerce was very helpful and accepting of me.

Another big challenge that I encountered involved travel. In order to progress professionally, I found that I needed to travel to conferences, classes and so on. I found it difficult to locate accessible transportation between airports and hotels, decent accessible hotel rooms, rental vehicles that could accommodate the wheelchair and other things I needed such as repair facilities when the airlines damaged my wheelchair. I encountered difficulty with some airlines in terms of following rules and transporting my wheelchair without breaking it. I took to traveling with a copy of the Air Carriers' Access Act, the law which delineates the rights of travelers with disabilities.

The thing that I always admired about you was the way you seemed to go a lot of places in the wheelchair and how it never seemed to stop you. Tell us about that and how this attitude helped you get ready to get well.

Maybe I'm not terribly bright, but I never understood the idea that a disability should stop a person from doing whatever he or she wants to do. I have always believed that people of good intentions will find a way over, under or around barriers. I guess this is what prevented me from feeling like I was a different person in the wheelchair than I had been before. I think that this attitude helped me to get ready to get well because I still felt like ME inside and I had not adopted the disability as a part of my personality. Even though I had some fears and did not know "Healthy Nancie" I knew the Nancie I had been. I had muscular dystrophy for years before the diagnosis, but I did not know it and I perceived myself as healthy but not very physical.

Can you remember the exact moment that you said "Now's the time." Can you share with us the process you went through at that time?

Yes. I was at a conference and I simply decided that I was going to do it. I was feeling annoyed at being in the wheelchair, like I said, which was new feeling for me. Somewhere deep inside of me I knew that I was ready, so I sought out the practitioner whose techniques, personality and abilities seemed the best match for my needs.

Is there anything that you can share with us about your process in the two days of cellular cleansing that would help other people?

The exact process of cellular cleansing is not really the important issue. People can choose from a plethora of practitioners and techniques, based on their individual needs and preferences. However, the process I went through inside of myself is relevant, and I think it's what you are asking. I went into the process with a belief that I would gain everything from it that I could, whatever that might be. I had decided that I was going to go along with the process as fully as I could, doing whatever I was asked to do to the best of my ability. I was a hypnotherapist but I was not going to try to control or second-guess the practitioner or her techniques, rather I decided to allow the change to occur.

Can you share with us some thoughts that can help others who may feel stuck in their own patterns but who want to get well?

Yes, and thanks so much for asking this question. I firmly believe that if a person wants to get well, he or she must loosen and remove as much of the stuff that is making that change difficult.

In general, a positive and accepting attitude is really beneficial when working with any new process or practitioner. Please allow yourself to believe and trust in whatever and whomever you have chosen to bring on your journey to the city of Wellness.

You must allow the process or practitioner a clear shot at the target, so to speak. Do not run from healer to healer to healer without letting any of it work unfettered by other practices. That is simply ineffective, expensive and unfair to yourself. I have seen several people do this and they don't get the benefit of whatever they chose to try. When I see this, I understand that this individual is not really ready to get rid of whatever stuff is there, and for whatever reason he or she is feeling like it must appear that there is effort to change the condition.

If I had to boil it down to one piece of advice, I would have to say, "Trust your body and your choices!"

Patti Conklin's Story

Patti Conklin was born in the late 1950s near Ithaca, NY. She was the third of four children. From an early age, Patti was extremely intelligent and verbal. She saw nonphysical beings as clearly as she saw her family and in fact did not know there was a difference when she was very young. She has told the story of discovering the difference when she attempted to hug a "friend" and her hand went right through their body.

Patti Conklin carries the gift and the burden of sight and sensitivity that are beyond, and different from, the normal five senses that other people experience. She does not see the world in a solid, physical way as most of us do. She sees the vibrations of the people and objects around her. If she looks at physical object such as a cup, for instance, she will see it as a semi-solid shape with a vibratory rate that is unique. A different object will have a different vibratory rate, and so she is able to distinguish objects and live beings because of the differences in their vibrations.

Patti has always been able to see into the human body, noticing energy flow and blockages. She is often able to identify the emotion or type of stuff that caused the blockage. Her interest in observing this allowed her to realize that energy blockages can cause illness and disease. Over time, she learned to manipulate energy to affect these blockages and help people heal themselves.

One thing that Patti noticed while observing people's speech was that the words affect only the speaker, not anyone else. It is impossible for anyone to say nasty things to another and cause that person to have a health problem or energy block. This is an important point, as it is a cornerstone of what Patti later taught and how she worked with individuals. It is also important for individuals who are ready to get rid of their stuff to understand that the words of other people in no way created their stuff, but rather their repeating and reacting to those words.

Throughout her life, Patti has had what she calls "visitations" from a voice she identifies as "Father" or "God." Since early childhood, she has experienced these visitations, as well as receiving information or instructions from this voice. She has always obeyed these instructions, courageously saying and doing what Father asks. It seems that many people receive instructions in this way, but it is rare for someone to obey unquestioningly as Patti does. Often people will say their "guidance" has told them to do what they really want to do anyway, but this is not true of Patti. Often she does not want to do what she is told by Father but she does it anyway, trusting that it will prove to be the right thing to do. This has served her well.

One of the most amazing things about Patti Conklin is her willingness and her ability to share her gift with others. She is very verbally skilled and is able to explain her vision to others and assist them in increasing their own intuitive abilities. She works with individuals and groups, both in educational workshops and in therapeutic settings.

A qualified hypnotherapist, Patti Conklin used these skills to develop specific techniques. These techniques utilize the skills of hypnosis and Neuro Linguistic Programming (NLP) as well as Patti's intuitive abilities. The most impressive and interesting of Patti's techniques is her "Cellular Cleansing" protocol.

Cellular Cleansing allows the individual to clear energy blockages quickly and efficiently. In approximately six to eight hours of work people can clear up to 70% of their stuff-created blockages. This can result in dramatic changes in wellness.

Well Again

Since my own experience with Cellular Cleansing, a myriad of wonderful things have happened for me. The first and most amazing is that I no longer have muscular dystrophy or any symptoms of my former medical problem. I have not used the wheelchair or other adaptive equipment since approximately April 13, 2003. I can walk as much as I want, dance, ride a bicycle, and do whatever I choose. I love to hear my family remind me that I am "cured" when I ask them to do something. I still insist that my family take on their fair share of household tasks and they are more than willing to do so. My wellness is a gift and I never forget that.

Professionally, I have had wonderful opportunities because of the Cellular Cleansing. In 2003, Patti Conklin chose to begin training associates to do the work she does, including Cellular Cleansing. In a conversation at my home in May of that year, I expressed interest in taking the training, which she agreed would be a good thing for me. I trained with Patti in July and October of 2003 and became one of her first Certified Associates. I began to offer workshops in her techniques and information, as well as Cellular Cleansings. It is a great treat to be able to help others as I was helped.

My own personal stuff related to judgment. I was incredibly judgmental of others, their actions, beliefs, and everything else about them. I had a great deal of critical mass stuff because of these judgments and attitudes, which I had begun to experience in the womb.

My mother is not a rude or unpleasant person in any way, but she does not suffer fools gladly, as they say. As is very common, in the womb I experienced her emotions as she dealt with the people around her who were for the most part less educated and worldly that she and my father were. From the stories she has told, I know my mother found the women in the town in which I was born to be different from her usual sorts of friends in ways that she found personally challenging. While I am sure that she was always polite, her inner emotions and judgments were going on inside her own body. These were passed on to me.

My judgmental feelings and emotions, which are naturally related to Fear and tend to cause anger, were lodged in my skeletal muscles. This caused the pain and fatigue with which I lived. In other words, I was dealing with Critical Mass stuff in the muscles of my body. I used massage therapy, acupuncture, shiatsu, and chiropractic care to loosen the stuff until it was the appropriate time to remove it with the Cellular Cleansing.

In addition, I had some Replay stuff going on which caused the common intestinal issues that people with mitochondrial myopathy can have. These symptoms are chronic diarrhea alternating with constipation. I remember being asked by a medical doctor at one time whether I still had control of my bowels, the loss of which was a horrific idea to me. To loosen this stuff, I saw a physical therapist for visceral manipulation until the Cellular Cleansing helped me to remove it.

I had little if any Free-Floating stuff. My immune system was reasonably good, and my general health was considered to be about average for my age, as long as the muscular dystrophy was factored out. However, since removing so much of all my stuff, I have noticed a difference. I used to get bronchitis at least annually, and this is no longer the case. It makes a nice and totally unexpected change.

Because I know that it was primarily judgment that got me into trouble, I monitor myself. I am careful not to judge others as I once did. It actually feels a lot better not to have those feelings and attitudes any more. Do I occasionally fall into old habits? You had better believe I do! However, it is something I generally notice and address with myself immediately. I regularly remove the judgment from my body because I notice some discomfort if I forget to do this. I am careful that, even if I feel a judgment, I do not speak it as my words enter my body only and can cause blockages, as we know. I am told that I am softer, gentler, kinder, and more unconditionally loving in my speech now. This is a good thing in my opinion. I am definitely not perfect, nor do I ever expect to be. I am just myself as I was born to be without the judgment, anger, and fear-based stuff that I do not need.

When you get rid of the majority of your stuff, you will feel better, act better, and speak more kindly. Whatever methods of loosening and eventually removing your stuff you choose, you will be glad you did. Your physical, mental, and emotional health will likely improve.

Please understand, however, that the changes may or may not be in the ways you expect or desire. Some physical conditions change dramatically for one individual and do not for another. This does NOT mean that you are undeserving or bad or did something rotten in a previous lifetime. It may be that you have not yet found the methods that will work best for removing your stuff from your individual body. It may mean that the condition in which you find yourself is one that you have unconsciously chosen for this lifetime, what some call the life lesson you came here to learn. Remember that there is no fault or blame in the stuff we carry. It is what it is, just stuff that you did not intentionally take on, at least not consciously.

We all have stuff. I have it, you have it, and the most highly evolved person on the planet has it. If we were 100% unstuffed, we would no longer be human. The goal is not to be totally rid of stuff, which is impossible anyway because we constantly gather little bits here and there as we go through our normal lives. We constantly take it on but well people constantly throw it off as well. The goal is to be as clear and unstuffed as is possible. In this way, we can be as well as is possible in all areas given our age and other normal considerations.

Resource List

MASSAGE AND BODYWORK

Therapist Referrals

American Massage Therapy Association
820 Davis Street
Evanston, IL 60201
www.amtamassage.org

Association of Massage and Bodywork Professionals
1271 Sugarbush Drive
Evergreen, Colorado 80439
www.abmp.com

Books and Materials

MOSBY's Fundamentals of Therapeutic Massage
Sandy Fritz, MS

Hands On Healing: Massage Remedies For Hundreds of Health Problems by the Editors of Prevention Magazine health Books
Edited by John Feltman

ACUPUNCTURE/ACUPRESSURE

Books and Materials

Acupuncture: How It Works, How It Cures
Peter Firebrace and Sandra Hill

Between Heaven and Earth
Efrem Korn and Harriet Beinfield

PROCESS ACUPRESSURE

Practitioner Referrals

Process Acupressure Unlimited
PO Box 1096
Capitola, CA 95010
(818) 464-4606
www.processacupressure.com

Books and Materials

Soul Return: Integrating Body, Psyche and Spirit
Aminah Raheem

ZERO BALANCING

Practitioner Referrals

The Zero Balancing Association
801 West Main Street, Suite 202
Charlottesville, VA 22903
(434) 244-2645

Books and Materials

Inner Bridges: A Guide toEnergy Movement and Body Structure
Fritz Frederick Smith

Zero Balancing: Touching the energy of The Bone
John Hamwee and Fritz Smith

SHIATSU

Practitioner Referrals

American Organization for Bodywork Therapies of Asia
1010 Haddonfield-Berlin Road, Suite 408
Voorhees, NJ 08043-3514
(856) 782-1616
www.aobta.org

Books and Materials

Contact the organization listed above for recommendations

EMOTIONAL FREEDOM TECHNIQUE

Practitioner Referrals

Emotional Freedom Techniques
Gary H, Craig
PO Box 1393
Gualala, CA 95445
www.emofree.com

Books and Materials

The EFT Manual
Gary Craig

Adventures in EFT
Silvia Hartmann

REIKI

Practitioner Referrals

The Reiki Alliance
204 N. Chestnut Street
Kellogg, ID 83837
(208) 783-3535

Books and Materials.

Contact the above organization for recommendations

TALK THERAPIES

Practitioner Referrals

American Psychological Association
750 First Street, NE
Washington, DC 20002-4242
www.apa.org

Books and Materials.

Contact the above organization for recommendations

COGNITIVE-BEHAVIORAL THERAPY

Practitioner Referrals

Association For the Advancement of Behavior Therapy
305 7th Ave, 16th Floor
New York, NY 10001
(212) 647-1890
www.aabt.org

Books and Materials.

Contact the above organization for recommendations

WESTERN MEDICINE

Practitioner Referrals
American Medical Association
515 North State Street
Chicago, IL 60610
(800) 621-8335
www.ama-assn.org

Books and Materials

Merck Manual: Diagnosis and Therapy
Robert Berkow, Mark H. Beers and Mark Burs

CHIROPRACTIC

Practitioner Referrals
International Chiropractors' Association
1110 North Glebe Road, Suite 1000
Arlington, VA 22201

Books and Materials

Chiropractic First by Terry A. Rondberg

CRANIO-SACRAL THERAPY

Practitioner Referrals

The Upledger Institute
11211 Prosperity Farms Road, D-325
Palm Beach Gardens, FL 33410-3487
(561) 622-4334
www.upledger.com

Books and Materials

Contact the Upledger Institute for reference materials.

VISCERAL MANIPULATION

Practitioner Referrals

The Upledger Institute
11211 Prosperity Farms Road, D-325
Palm Beach Gardens, FL 33410-3487
(561) 622-4334
www.upledger.com

Books and Materials

Contact the Upledger Institute for reference materials.

HYPNOTHERAPY

Practitioner Referrals

International Association of Counselors and Therapists
10915 Bonita Beach Road, Suite 1101
Bonita Springs, FL 34135
(239) 498-9710
www.iact.org

International Hypnosis Federation
30819 Casilina Drive
Rancho Palos Verdes, CA 90275
(310) 541-4844
www.hypnosisfederation.com

National Association of Transpersonal Hypnotherapists
PO Box 249
Goshen, VA 24439
(800) 296-MIND
www.holistictree.com

American Board of Hypnotherapy
615 Piikoi Street, Suitc 501
Honolulu, HI 96814
(800) USA-9996
www.hypnosis.com

Books and Materials

The Wizard Within
A.M. Krasner

My Voice Will Go With You: The Teaching Tales of Milton Erickson
Ernest Rossi

MEDICAL INTUITION

Practitioner Referrals

Patti L. Conklin
Healing Within
PO Box 870909
Stone Mountain, GA 30087
(888) 376-3301
www.patticonklin.com

Books and Materials

The Book of Miracles
Josie Ravenwing

UNSTUFFING YOURSELF

Practitioner Referrals

Dr. Nancie M. Barwick
10807 Main Street, Suite 600
Fairfax, VA 22030
(703) 385-9311
www.doctornancie.com

Books and Materials

Beyond Disability: Toward Self Acceptance and Peace
Nancie M. Barwick

Index

B

C

T